DATE DUE

MAR - 3 1995	
OCT 2 0 1995	
OCT 3 1 1995	
NOV 2 9 199:	
DEC 1 1 1995	
MAR 1 1 1996	
NOV 2 7 1996	
MAR 3 1997	
DEC - 4 2000	

BRODART   Cat. No. 23-221

FEDERALISM AND HEALTH POLICY

The Development of Health Systems in
Canada and Australia

Canada is at present one of the most decentralized operative federations
while Australia is one of the most centralized. Using the development of
health care in the respective systems as models, Gwendolyn Gray examines the validity of competing theories of federalism.

Orthodox theories contend that a federal division of power restricts the
expansion of the democratic state and results in weak, conservative government. In contrast, the 'revisionist' theories, which have emerged recently
in Canada, argue that federalism contributes to the growth of governments
and may, under favourable circumstances, facilitate innovative policy development.

Gray suggests that the way federal institutions function depends on the
particular set of arrangements in operation at a given time and on the complex interaction of historical, social, economic, and political factors. If this
is so, she concludes, the search for a theory of federalism with universal validity is likely to be a futile exercise.

GWENDOLYN GRAY is a member of the Department of Political Science at the
Australian National University.

GWENDOLYN GRAY

Federalism and Health Policy: The Development of Health Systems in Canada and Australia

UNIVERSITY OF TORONTO PRESS
Toronto Buffalo London

© University of Toronto Press 1991
Toronto Buffalo London
Printed in Canada

ISBN 0-8020-5904-X (cloth)
ISBN 0-8020-6862-6 (paper)

Printed on acid-free paper

Canadian Cataloguing in Publication Data

Gray, Gwendolyn
    Federalism and health policy

    Includes bibliographical reference and index.
    ISBN 0-8020-5904-X (bound) ISBN 0-8020-6862-6 (pbk.)

    1. Medical policy – Canada. 2. Medical policy – Australia.
    3. Insurance, Health – Canada. 4. Insurance, Health –
    Australia. 5. Federal government – Canada. 6. Federal
    government – Australia. I. Title.

    RA412.5.C3G7 1991   368.4′2′00971 C91-094282-X

This book has been published with the help of a grant from Hollinger Inc.

To my mother, Ethel Agreta Swan

Contents

viii Contents

List of Tables

Abbreviations

AMA	Australian Medical Association
AMG	*Australasian Medical Gazette*
BCMA	British Columbia Medical Association
BMA	British Medical Association
CCF	Cooperative Commonwealth Federation
CLSC	Les centres locaux de services communautaires (local community service centres)
CMA	Canadian Medical Association
CPD	*Commonwealth Parliamentary Debates*
CPI	Consumer Price Index
CRSSS	Les Conseils régionaux de la santé et des services sociaux (Regional Councils for Health and Social Services)
DSC	Les départéments de santé communautaire (Departments of Community Health)
EPF	Established-Programs Financing
FLQ	Front de Libération du Québec
FMOQ	Fédération des médicins omnipracticiens du Québec (Federation of General Medical Practitioners of Quebec)
FMSQ	Fédération des médicins spécialistes du Québec (Federation of Medical Specialists of Quebec)
GNP	Gross National Product
HACC	Home and Community Care Program
HHSC	Hospitals and Health Services Commission (Australia)
HR	House of Representatives
JCSS	Joint Committee on Social Security
KODC	Keep Our Doctors Committee

MMA   Manitoba Medical Association
MJA   *Medical Journal of Australia*
NDP   New Democratic Party
NHMRC National Health and Medical Research Council
OMA   Ontario Medical Association
PQ   Parti Québécois
QHIB   Quebec Health Insurance Board

Preface

Australian federalism was the subject of a significant revival of interest in the 1970s. Each of the major parties developed 'new federalism' policies that reflected divergent views about the appropriate role of the state, especially in areas of social policy. The use of the extensive constitutional and financial powers that had accrued to the Commonwealth after 1900 became a highly controversial issue when an interventionist Labor government came to power in 1972. In keeping with Labor tradition, the Whitlam government attempted, during its three years in office, to enhance the power and prestige of the Commonwealth. At the same time, federal responsibility for new and existing social policies and programs was increased substantially. Gough Whitlam argued that only the federal government had the capacity to effectively promote equality; accordingly, the major functions of society should therefore be 'hitched to the star of the Commonwealth.'

During their sojourn in opposition, the non-Labor parties developed their own 'new federalism,' partly as a response to the centralization of the Whitlam period. The Liberal commitment to the preservation of a federal system was reaffirmed as a means of providing 'an effective barrier against centralist, authoritarian control' and against the growth of 'socialism.' The stated aims of the new federalism were to decentralize power and to return revenue and policy responsibility to the level of government 'closest to the people.' It soon became apparent, however, that, although the Fraser government aimed to minimize Commonwealth responsibility in a number of social-policy areas, it did not intend to transfer financial power to the states. Under these circumstances, the states were unlikely to expand their activities in areas from which the federal government had withdrawn. 'New federalism' was therefore an important element in the social-policy strategies of both major parties.

The original aim of this study was to explore the relationship between federalism, ideology, and social-policy development in Australia. During the course of my research, an opportunity arose to attend a conference in Alberta on Canada's national health-care system. Papers presented at the conference and discussions with participants provided insights into the processes of policy making in a much more decentralized federation. Canadian experience suggested that many of the assumptions widely held in Australia about the impact of federalism on the scope of government activity needed to be re-examined. Consequently, I decided that it would be a worthwhile exercise to undertake a comparative study of the development of Canadian and Australian health policy.

To the many people who helped me in a variety of ways in the preparation of this book, I express my sincere appreciation. In particular, I would like to thank Canadian policy makers and analysts for the time, information, and documents they so generously gave me in 1985, often at very short notice. More than forty people made themselves available for formal interviews and many others made time for informal discussions. I am grateful, too, for the generous hospitality I was shown all over Canada. Australian policy makers and experts were equally helpful, and I thank them sincerely. Among the people who read parts or all of the manuscript and offered comments are David Adams, Brian Galligan, John Ballard, Pat Weller, and John Deeble. In particular, the assistance of David Adams and Brian Galligan was invaluable. John Hart and Marian Sawer offered encouragement. The manuscript was typed by Sharon Merton and corrected cheerfully and efficiently by Sharon Merton and Judy Robson, and Sue Fraser's editorial assistance was superb. My thanks to Virgil Duff of University of Toronto Press who shepherded the manuscript through the many processes necessary for publication. Last, but not least, I thank my children, Bridget, Brendan, and Sophia, and my husband, John, for their understanding and help.

Gwen Gray
December 1990

FEDERALISM AND HEALTH POLICY

Introduction

In the last two hundred years, a large and influential literature has accumulated on the operation of federal systems of government. Although diverse, this literature is dominated by a frequently recurring theme: that the division of economic, constitutional, and political power among the constituent units of a polity operates to restrict the exercise of political power. Under such a system of division, the extent to which government can intervene effectively in economic and social life is held to be severely constrained. Social democrats have thus criticized the system, which, they argue, operates to preserve the status quo, militating against the formulation of appropriate policy responses to changing economic, social, and political conditions. In contrast, many advocates of 'small' government support a federal division of power as a means of curtailing expansion. It is widely held, then, that federalism acts as a barrier to change. A recent study of the development of social policy in Canada found evidence to support such a view: federalism first slowed the expansion of the welfare state, and then, in the 1980s, operated to protect social programs from those who would dismantle them (Banting 1987).

Theories of federalism therefore identify institutional factors as major determinants of government activity and public-policy outcomes. Institutions are central not only to traditional federalism theories but also to a strand of thinking that has emerged in recent years and is termed a 'revisionist' theory. In this view, federalism facilitates the growth of government and the range of its activities, primarily because it multiplies the governmental units that operate in a given jurisdiction. Surprisingly, few analysts have questioned the validity of the main arguments of this body of thought, even though modern policy studies have shown that a multitude of factors interact together through institutional structures to influence the scope and shape of government outputs. Other identified policy determinants include levels of economic development, ideas and ideologies, interest-group activities, and partisan political competition, to name just a few. Theories that attribute major explanatory power to a single variable such as federalism must therefore be subject to considerable doubt.

The problems that attend concentrating on federal arrangements in preference to other policy influences that may be at least equally important are compounded by the 'slippery' nature of the meaning of the term 'federalism,' which is both a relative and a dynamic concept. It is a relative concept because most countries have some degree of division of power among orders or institutions of government; many unitary countries, for example, have strong local government. It is a dynamic concept because federalism is highly political, and balances of power are rarely static, despite the rigidity of written constitutions. Moreover, the institutions of federalism vary enormously, both by county and by historical eras within a county.

Even a cursory glance at two federations such as Canada and Australia, which otherwise share many common characteristics, uncovers illustrations of these points. First, political, financial, and constitutional powers are far more decentralized in Canada than in Australia, a set of arrangements that appears to reflect Canada's greater cultural, economic, and linguistic diversity. Canada is thus a 'more federal' nation than Australia. Second, the balance of power in both countries has changed dramatically over time but the pattern and direction of change have been quite different. Canada has alternated between periods of centralization and decentralization, with the overall trend to date being towards decentralization. In contrast, there has been a steady, incremental movement towards centralization throughout Australia's federal history. Third, many of the institutions of federalism differ in a number of ways and develop and change over time. For example, the Australian constitution provided for domestic amendment by referendum from the beginning whereas the Canadian constitution could be amended only by the British Parliament until repatriation in 1982. Moreover, whereas judicial interpretation has generally taken a narrow view of the federal government's powers in Canada, since 1920 the reverse has been the case in Australia. Another important difference that affects national government power is the fact that Canada's Senate is appointed whereas Australia's is elected. Australian governments often do not control the Upper House, and pieces of legislation, including money bills, can be and have been blocked. Institutional procedures for the coordination of federal financial arrangements are also markedly different. For example, where Australia established a loans council in 1928 to coordinate government borrowing, no formal coordinating mechanism has been set up in Canada. Canada relies on ministerial conferences and intergovernmental negotiations to determine equalization grants to the provinces whereas an independent body, the Australian Grants Commission, was established for that purpose in 1933.

Thus, the term 'federalism' has no clearly defined or precise meaning. To describe a political system as a federation tells us very little about the distribution of political power, the institutions of federalism, or the dynamics of the system. And it tells us nothing about a range of other forces that have been shown to be important determinants of public policy.

The aim of this book is to re-examine theories of federalism using evidence from case-studies of policy formulation in two federations. As Leslie (1987: 43) argues, 'it is, ultimately, the knowledge obtained through case studies that will enable one to make an informed judgement about the impact of federalism on policy – its alleged conservatism, the extent to which it augments the political power of regional elites ... and so forth.' The case-studies will be set in historical perspective in order to take account of federal dynamics and to examine the effects of changes over time. Some of the questions that will be addressed are whether federalism indeed impedes the growth of government and creates structural barriers against change and whether federal systems are always characterized by intergovernmental conflict and jurisdictional disputes that promote delays and deadlocks. Is it possible, perhaps, that intergovernmental conflict and competition can sometimes lead to policy expansion? Does federalism enhance the power of interest groups by multiplying the number of access points to decision-making processes? Is the centralization of power a necessary precondition for the introduction of social-democratic reforms, as the Australian Labor party has always argued, or can innovations sometimes be made equally well in a decentralized system? Is federal government weak and conservative? Or is it the case, as we might predict from public-policy analysis, that the way federal systems operate depends on the particular federation in question at a given time and on a complex interaction between federal institutions and the many other influences that shape government action and public-policy outcomes?

The two federations chosen for study are Canada and Australia. These countries share many economic, cultural, and institutional similarities, which makes them suitable subjects for comparison because fewer variables need to be fed into the analysis. At the same time, the important differences in federal arrangements will enable comparisons to be made of the impact of different degrees of centralization and decentralization.

Health is the policy area selected for detailed examination. It is a particularly appropriate area for a study of the influences and constraints on policy development because there are usually both costs and benefits associated with government intervention. On the one hand, health policies are expensive and place large and often unpredictable burdens on government budgets. Powerful interest groups, particularly organized medicine, are active in the area, and strong ideological differences about the appropriate form and extent of government intervention are common. On the other hand, policies that reduce financial barriers to access to health services are popular and have often been an ingredient in electoral success. Finally, health provides an opportunity to study the impact of federal arrangements because, in both Canada and Australia, constitutional responsibility for the provision of services is divided between federal and regional governments.

This study is organized as follows: the first chapter examines briefly the main ideas of orthodox theories of federalism and of public-policy analysis. It then outlines the similarities and differences between Canada and Australia and charts changes in the federal balances of power, including changes in constitutional responsibility for the provision of health care. Chapter 2 traces the development of Canada's national health-insurance system. In chapter 3, the Australian tradition of direct service provision, which culminated in an attempt to introduce a national health service along British lines in the 1940s, is examined. The implementation of voluntary health insurance, the Australian medical profession's preferred policy, is outlined in chapter 4. Chapter 5 examines the highly controversial cost-containment policies of Canadian governments after the introduction of Medicare and the abolition of direct charges to patients in the mid-1980s. The implementation of national health insurance in Australia is the subject of chapter 6. In chapter 7, recent innovations in the organization of the health-care delivery systems in both countries are compared and contrasted. The case-study evidence is then used in chapter 8 to identify the main determinants of policy development and to examine and assess the role of federal institutions.

1

Federalism and the Study
of Public Policy

'Federalism' is a term used to describe sets of arrangements that vary enormously – in formal structure, in actual operation, and over time. Consequently, it is a term that scholars have found very difficult to define. Classical definitions of federalism emphasize the legal and institutional aspects of the system. Wheare (1953: 11), for example, defined the 'federal principle' as 'the method of dividing powers so that the general and regional governments are each, within a sphere, coordinate and independent.' According to this definition, only the United States, Australia, and Switzerland are true federations (Wheare 1953: 16–34). Reagan (1972: 10–11) has argued that even the United States fails to qualify on this definition because the federal government can, in practice, legislate in any sphere with the result that there is no area reserved exclusively for the states. Similarly, Australia can no longer be called a true federation because the financial dominance of the Commonwealth has eroded the independence of the states.

In the 1950s, the descriptive value of legal definitions of federalism came into question. Such definitions were seen as static and rigid, offering only limited information and making no allowance for change. In response to perceived shortcomings, there emerged what has been termed a 'dynamic' concept of federalism (Wiltshire 1986: 69–70). In a much-quoted article, Livingston (1967: 37) argued that 'the essence of federalism lies not in the institutional or constitutional structure but in society itself. Federal government is a device by which the federal qualities of society are articulated and protected.' He went on to contend that federalism is a relative rather than absolute term and that societies should be seen as ranging along a spectrum from 'theoretically wholly integrated' at one extreme to 'theoretically wholly diversified' at the other (1967:

43–5). Davies (1964: 61–4) put forward a similar case, arguing that 'federalness is only a matter of degree.' Typical of the dynamic perspective is the argument that 'enduring federalism is not static and merely constitutional. It is dynamic and often unstable. It is highly political and is ultimately rooted in territorially-oriented, social and cultural diversity' (Hodgins and Wright 1978: 289–90).

Adequate definitions or descriptions of federalism thus need to be able to accommodate the reality of change. However, the notion that federalism is a product of societies rather than of governments has been questioned recently by two Canadian writers. Cairns (1977) has suggested that powerful, independent regional governments may be the product of governmental élites rather than of underlying sociological forces. Similarly, Simeon (1977: 297) has argued that governments, once established, 'come to shape and influence the environment.' The difficulties involved in arriving at comprehensive descriptions and explanations of the disparate and changing sets of relationships found in modern federations have led one eminent writer to consider as 'futile' attempts to define 'either the word or the thing.' Instead, G. Sawer (1976: 2) speaks of a very loose 'federal situation' 'where geographical division of the power to govern is desired or has been achieved in a way giving the several governmental units of the system some degree of security – some guarantee of continued existence as organisations and as holders of power.'

Despite the variety of approaches, most writers include the concept of a division of power as one of the essential elements of a federal system (Diamond 1963: 25). And it is the division of the power of the state that is held to have a profound impact on government activity and on policy outcomes.

Theories of Federalism

The theories of federalism considered here are divided into two broad groupings on the basis of the very different sets of claims that are made about the impact of federal institutions. The theories in the first group are termed 'orthodox.' They hold to the conventional position, first articulated by James Madison, that a federal division of power is a means of controlling the use (and possible abuse) of political power. The second group of theories is labelled 'revisionist' because they overturn most of the arguments of the 'orthodox' school. In this view, federalism is characterized by expansionist tendencies that promote the growth of government and the range of its activities.

The distinction between 'orthodox' and 'revisionist' theories follows the approach taken by Banting (1982, 1987) and Leslie (1987: 41–4). This distinction, it needs to be acknowledged, is achieved at some cost to the complexities and nuances of many of the arguments. Moreover, not all writers have been prepared to make broad claims about the impact of federalism: some students have argued that the effects of the system vary according to the interaction of institutions with a range of other forces and influences, such as particular policy areas and the federal balance of power at any given time. Writers who have taken the view that the nature of federalism is contingent on other factors include Elazar (1962), Leman (1977), Tuohy (1989a), and some members of the public-choice school, particularly Ostrom (1969, 1973, 1987) and Sproule-Jones (1975). Nevertheless, attempts to develop theories of federalism that have general validity are common, and the distinction between 'orthodox' and 're-visionist' approaches is very useful because it serves to identify two of the major strands of thinking in the literature.

Orthodox Theories

James Madison, one of the founders of the first modern federation, the United States, believed that no man or group of men, either populist leaders or popular majorities, could be trusted with unlimited power. The preservation of individual rights and the property-holding rights of the minority required that the use of political power be checked on all sides (Madison 1961: 129–36). Federalism was one of the principal means by which the power of government was to be 'structured, channelled and moderated' in the new republic. Therefore, representative rather than direct democracy was instituted. Power was then divided, first between the federal and the state governments, and then between the institutions of each government. As Madison explained the system in *Federalist* 51, 'in the compound republic of America, the power surrendered by the people is first divided between two distinct governments and then the portion allotted to each subdivided among distinct and separate departments. Hence, a double security arises to the rights of the people. The different governments will control each other at the same time that each will be controlled by itself' (1961: 357–8).

This fragmentation of power would also contain the spread of radical movements. Madison argued that 'a rage for paper money, for an abolition of debts, for an equal division of property, or for any other improper or wicked project, will be less apt to pervade the whole body of the Union than a particular member of it; in the same proportion as such a malady is more likely to taint a particular county or district than an entire state' (1961: 136).

Writing in 1984, Lowi argued that the American system of government has worked just as the founders intended. He concluded that institutional arrangements are the main reason that socialism does not exist as a significant political force. The distribution of power among a number of governments has produced a form of 'Balkanization,' which means that interests can dominate in one part of the country without being able to spread by means of majority rule. The limited functions of the national government for the first one hundred and fifty years after federation meant that there was 'no national pattern of law, legitimation or repression to confirm a socialist critique.' The cities functioned as localizing agents, and the states have been, and remain, 'bastions of conservatism.' Because the American national state has expanded, Lowi argues, socialism is more likely to emerge as a political force in future (1984: 369–80).

Federalism has been defended on the grounds that, under such a system, political oppression is less likely to emerge than it is in a unitary state;[1] that it protects minority rights and permits cultural, linguistic, religious, and ideological diversity; and that it 'combines the economic advantages of large size with the possibilities for self-government that exist in a smaller political community' (Stevenson 1979: 20–4). However, in the last hundred years, a growing body of literature has emerged that accepts the main arguments of the 'orthodox' position and is critical of federalism as a system of government. One of the first and most often quoted anti-federalists is English constitutionalist A.V. Dicey. His focus reflects nineteenth-century changes in ideas about the appropriate role of the democratic state.

Critiques of Federalism

Dicey argued that federalism gives rise to weak, conservative, legalistic government. The division of the power of the sovereign state tends to 'limit on every side the action of government.' Written constitutions that cannot be amended easily place constraints on both central and regional governments, and judges charged with constitutional interpretation become 'masters' of the constitution. Dicey acknowledged that some people support limited government but recorded that it was not favoured by the democrats of his day. Federalism maintains 'the status quo in politics,' he argued, and is therefore 'incompatible with schemes for wide social innovation' (1959: 138–80).

Conflict over the most appropriate policies to deal with the problems of the depression of the 1930s brought forth both federal and anti-federal responses in America. In a paper entitled 'The Obsolescence of Federalism,' Harold Laski argued that 'the problems of dual occupancy of the same ground hinders at every turn the creative solutions of the problems involved unless we conceive of those solutions in terms of geological time' (1939: 308).

Another important argument about the constraining effects of federalism is that it enhances the power of interest groups. By multiplying the number of actors, the number of decision points, and the number of veto points, federalism provides groups with many opportunities to influence public policy. Governments can be played off against each other, and groups can concentrate their efforts at the level of government most likely to be receptive to their aims. The argument is sometimes made that groups are more likely to be successful at the provincial or state level of government (Key 1952: 102; Wilenski 1983: 87–9; Laski 1939: 308; Porter 1965: 380–1, 384–5). Grodzins (1967: 268) has termed this the 'multiple-crack' attribute of American government. 'Multiple-crack,' he argues, has two meanings: first, there are 'many fissures or access points,' and second, and 'less statically,' there are 'opportunities for wallops and smacks at government.' Pressman and Wildavsky's (1973) study of the difficulties that surrounded the implementation of a federal employment-generating program in the United States found support for these ideas, and support has also been found in some Canadian studies, although contrary evidence also exists (Smiley 1980: 148–53). There are no detailed studies of the implications of federal structures for interest-group activity in Australia.

In summary, while federalists and anti-federalists of the 'orthodox' school disagree about the value of federalism, they are in substantial agreement that the system constrains the scope of government activity. Wheare summarized the general orthodoxy in a paper delivered to an Australian Jubilee seminar in 1951: 'the fact is that the federal form of constitution involves certain restrictions upon governments which prevent the will of a majority in legislatures or a majority of the people from being carried out and it is the existence of these obstacles and restrictions which people find hard to accept. These restrictions are inseparable from federalism; they are indeed an expression of its nature ... Federal constitutions are classified by political scientists as rigid; they exhibit judicial review; they are legalistic and conservative' (Wheare 1951, quoted in Wilenski 1983: 84–5).

Few students of federalism would deny, of course, that there are other important influences on government and on public-policy development, but, for the most part, the question of what these forces are and how they interact with federal institutions is not addressed. However, implicit in the 'orthodox' view is the idea that a federal division of power will result in certain predictable outcomes, irrespective of the institutional forms adopted and of the social, political, and economic contexts of particular federations.

'Revisionist' Theories

In the 1960s and 1970s there emerged what Banting (1982: 73–7; 1987: 73–5) terms a 'revisionist' theory of federalism. This body of work is small, and the extent to which it can be said to constitute a theory of federalism, as distinct from a theory of Canadian federalism, might be questioned. However, it does present a challenge to time-honoured ideas from the 'orthodox' school.

'Revisionist' ideas are largely the work of two writers, Pierre Trudeau (1968) and Alan Cairns (1977, 1979). Both draw their arguments from observations of the operation of the Canadian system, and, although Trudeau makes generalizations about federalism, Cairns does not. However, writers outside Canada have also argued that there is inherent in federalism an expansionist dynamic. This literature is surveyed by Cameron (1978) in his examination of various explanations of the expansion of the public economy, which include an institutional explanation. The institutional explanation has two strands. First, federalism creates 'multiple, independent centres of public authority' (Cameron 1978: 1248). Writers such as Downs (1964), Niskanen (1971), Wildavsky (1974), and Heclo (1974), and neo-conservative writers such as Friedman and Friedman (1980), argue that bureaucracies have a proclivity to expand continuously. It follows that the more bureaucracies there are, the greater will be the growth of government and of government programs. The second strand in the institutional explanation is that public spending is likely to expand more rapidly in systems where the central financial authority has less than full control of the purse-strings. Cameron (1978: 1249) surveys a number of studies that conclude that public spending increases fastest at subnational levels of government. While unitary systems may also be decentralized, federalism is the arrangement most likely to produce fiscal and institutional decentralization.[2]

Banting (1982, 1987) finds that the arguments put forward by Cairns are consistent with these ideas. He observes that these arguments are also consistent with cross-national studies of welfare expenditure that show that federal systems spend less on social policy than do unitary systems. Taken together, Banting considers therefore that this disparate body of work constitutes a 'revisionist theory' of federalism.

Trudeau (1968) argues that federalism facilitates the expansion of government intervention in economic and social life. Radical policies can be more easily introduced in a federation than in a unitary system. Because the regions of a nation are always at different levels of political, social, and economic development, radical parties are likely to come to power in some jurisdictions but not in others. Socialist policies can then be introduced in parts of the country from which the 'seed of radicalism' can slowly spread. In unitary systems, innovation has to be delayed until a national consensus emerges. It would be a different matter, Trudeau argues, if all Canadians supported socialism. Socialist governments would then be elected in all jurisdictions and radical policies would be implemented 'no matter what the form of the constitution.' However, 'in a non-revoluntionary society ... no manner of reform can be implemented with sudden universality. Democratic reformers must proceed step-by-step ... The drive towards power must begin with the establishment of bridgeheads since at the outset it is obviously easier to convert specific groups or localities than to win over an absolute majority of the whole nation' (Trudeau 1968: 127).

In Trudeau's view, sovereignty is not weakened when it is divided. Rather, 'the sum total of governments has the sum total of powers.' Although there had been conflict and encroachment by one level of government on the jurisdiction of the other, Trudeau argues that, in practice, the history of Canadian federalism is one of 'intergovernmental exchange and cooperation.' Each level of government has an important role to play. What is needed, in Trudeau's opinion, is that responsibilities should be clarified so that citizens can demand 'good laws' from all governments (Trudeau 1968: 147–50).

Cairns's analysis is quite different from that of Trudeau but it shares the idea that a number of activist governments can coexist in a federation. Cairns argues that it is unnecessary to search for a sociological explanation for the enduring vitality of provincial regimes. The federal system creates multiple sets of bureaucratic and political élites that are possessed of tenacious instincts for their own preservation and growth' and endowed with 'an impressive array of jurisdictional financial, administrative and political resources.' All these units need to achieve their objectives is passivity or indifference from the electorate (Cairns 1979: 695–705).

In Cairns's view, the governments of Canada compete with each other for prestige and electoral support. This competition contributes to the growth of government and to the increasing impact of government on society, a trend that he argues created a crisis of overgovernment in the 1970s. Expansionism is further promoted because jurisdictional responsibilities are not clearly defined. The result is overlap and duplication. Moreover, the competitive struggle between governments results in a situation where every available policy area is occupied: 'slackness by one level of government provides the occasion for a preemptive strike by the other' (Cairns 1977: 189).

Both 'revisionist' and 'orthodox' ideas about the operation of federations will be examined below through the evidence from studies of health-policy development. We turn now to an examination of the main features of the Canadian and Australian federations. The very different directions in which the two systems have developed are traced briefly, and their main similarities and the differences between them are identified.

Two Federations

It has been argued recently that 'there are few countries in the world which have as much in common as Canada and Australia' (Symons 1982: 10). Both countries are geographically large and are well-endowed with natural resources, and both have relatively small populations. Levels of economic development and patterns of population dispersion are similar. Table 1 shows a number of selected Australian and Canadian statistics for 1986.

While there was a significant difference in 1986 rates of inflation, there was a remarkable similarity between average wages, currency values, and per-capita incomes. Thus, differences in levels of economic development, one of the major variables identified as influencing public policy, can be largely disregarded.

In institutional arrangements, too, there are strong similarities. Both countries have combined federalism with many of the institutions of parliamentary democracy, and strong, disciplined political parties have emerged. Policies designed to equalize the financial capacities of the states and provinces have been implemented. These similarities again limit the

TABLE 1
General data: Canada and Australia

	Canada	Australia
Population	25.3 million	15.7 million
Area	3.85 million sq.ml	3.00 million sq.m
Exchange rate	1 pound sterling	1 pound sterling
(February 1986)	= $C1.96	= $A1.94
Price Inflation	4.4 per cent	8.2 per cent
Approximate average wage	$C22,106 p.a.	$A21,450 p.a.
Per-capita income	$12,783	$13,600
Unemployment rate	10.2 per cent	7.4 per cent

SOURCE: Derived from Mercer (1986: 10, 37)

number of different variables that need to be compared. And in culture and education, there is 'a large measure of common heritage' and 'similar experience' (Symons 1982: 10).

In at least three respects, however, Canada and Australia are significantly different. As mentioned above, Australia does not share with Canada the characteristic of cultural dualism. This difference is one of the factors frequently put forward as at least part of the explanation for the trend towards decentralization in Canada and the reverse trend in Australia (Hodgins and Wright 1978: 289–304). A third major and related difference is in attitudes towards federalism. As we will see below, students of the subject and political actors view the institutions of divided power from quite different perspectives. Before examining these contrasting attitudes and ideas, however, we need to look a little more closely at the way the two systems have developed over time.

The Evolution of Canadian Federalism

The founders of the Canadian federation deliberately created a highly centralized system of government. They believed that one of the causes of civil war in the United States had been the independence of the states from central-government control. This problem and others were to be avoided by strong central government and by a restricted franchise (Hodgins 1978: 3–16, 43–5; Jones 1978: 19–41). The British North America Act of 1867 provided each level of government with control over a set of enumerated matters. The Dominion's powers encompassed all the functions of government that were important at the time and included the residual powers. The Dominion was assigned unlimited taxation powers whereas the provinces' powers were restricted to the field of direct taxation (Scott 1977: 292–3). Moreover, the Dominion had power to disallow provincial legislation, even in areas of exclusive provincial jurisdiction. It appointed provincial governors who could reserve bills for possible disallowance by the federal executive.

The Dominion, therefore, was in a dominant position. Because of these 'substantial modifications of the federal principle,' Wheare (1953: 19–21) classified Canada as a 'quasi-federal' system. Mallory (1977: 20) argues further that the original relationship resembled mother country and colony. However, these 'quasi-imperial' arrangements did not endure. Mallory identifies four later stages or 'faces' of Canadian development: classical, emergency, cooperative, and double-image federalism. While there is no clear distinction among these forms, they do fit roughly into historical periods.

Until 1949 the Judicial Committee of the Privy Council, composed of members of the British House of Lords, was the final appellate body for constitutional interpretation. According to Hogg (1985: 88–9), the process of judicial interpretation was dominated by two figures: Lord Watson from 1880 to 1899, and Lord Haldane from 1911 to 1929. Both men 'believed strongly in provincial rights and they established precedents which elevated the Provinces to coordinate status with the Dominion' (Hogg 1985: 89). The general powers of the federal government to legislate for the 'Peace, Order and Good Government' and for the regulation of trade and commerce were interpreted narrowly, whereas the power of the provinces to legislate in the area of 'Property and Civil Rights' was interpreted broadly, as were their powers of direct taxation (Smiley 1980: 31–41).

During the two world wars, the federal government assumed a range of powers that were normally the domain of the provinces. This move to 'emergency federalism' was supported by the courts. The peacetime distribution of powers was overridden, and, in effect, Canada became a unitary state. The emergency doctrine was abandoned, however, on return to peacetime conditions (Mallory 1977: 23–4).

Following the Second World War, judicial interpretation declined in importance as a determinant of the constitutional balance of power (Smiley 1980: 37–8). However, after the Supreme Court of Canada became the final court of appeal in 1949, the precedents established by the Judicial Committee were largely preserved, although there has been 'some growth of federal power' (Hogg 1985: 89). At the same time, changes took place that led to a form of 'cooperative federalism.' Under this mode of operation, both levels of government 'nominally' retained 'separate jurisdictions over different aspects of the same subject' but many policies were the result of joint decision-making processes. In addition to close and frequent consultation at both the officer and the ministerial level, cooperation took place through the delegation of regulatory functions to the provinces and through federal financial support for programs in provincial jurisdiction (Mallory 1977: 24–6).

Mallory argues that 'cooperative federalism' reduced provincial autonomy by distorting regional priorities. A reaction began in the mid-1960s that gave rise to a phase of 'double-image' federalism. This movement was led by Quebec in its determination to modernize, to assert its autonomy, and to preserve its cultural identity. It was reinforced when other provinces began to take a more activist role in economic and social policy and to demand greater control over revenue and spending decisions. Thus, the term 'double-image' federalism is used to describe a period of heightened provincial demands for independence. However, like many other phrases coined to try to describe various federal arrangements, it has no clearly definable meaning.

The historical evolution of Canadian federalism has been summarized by Watts as 'the cumulative impact of the interaction of Canada's federal institutions with the underlying social, economic and political forces would seem to have been the development not only of a stronger national community but also, concurrently, the growth of stronger provincial communities than existed in 1867. The net effect, despite the original quasi-federal centralist character of the British North America Act of 1867, has been a political system which now functions fundamentally in a fully coordinate federal manner' (1982: 20–1).

The Evolution of Australian Federalism

The Australian founders, unlike their Canadian counterparts, did not intend to create a strong national government. Instead, the federal government was invested primarily with those powers that were thought to be necessary to achieve common economic and defence objectives (Davies 1964: 59–61). A number of shared or concurrent powers were enumerated in Section 51 in such areas as trade and commerce, taxation, insurance, railways, postal and telegraphic services, conciliation and arbitration, marriage, and old-age and invalid pensions. The Commonwealth was given exclusive power in only a very few areas, such as customs and excise. The residual powers, by implication, were to rest with the states, which took over the constitutions, laws, and responsibilities of the former colonial governments, subject only to the limits of the new constitution. In the event of conflicting legislation in areas of concurrent power, Section 109 provides that federal law shall prevail. Disagreements were to be referred to the High Court. According to Wheare's definition, the Australian constitution of 1900 is 'clearly an example of a federal constitution' (Wheare 1953: 17).

In the early years, a dual, coordinate federal system operated (Mathews 1976: 8–12; Sawer 1977c: 5). By the 1920s, however, the federal balance had begun to change. One of the reasons was that the role of the Commonwealth had been expanded by the Labor government between 1910 and 1913. As in Canada, there was a growth of federal activity during the First World War. According to one writer, this activity had lasting implications through changed public attitudes towards the Commonwealth government (McMinn 1979: 135).

At the same time, a key change took place in judicial interpretation. Previous High Court decisions were criticized and overruled in the *Engineers'* case of 1920. This event ushered in a period that lasted until 1942 in which the powers of the Commonwealth were interpreted broadly. In the 1920s and 1930s, institutions were created for cooperative decision making in financial matters. A financial agreement was signed in 1927, the Loans Council was set up in 1928, and the first specific-purpose, conditional grants were made to the states. The High Court upheld the power of the Commonwealth to make grants in areas of state jurisdiction and to attach detailed conditions about the way the funds were to be spent. Thus, between the wars, 'coordinate' federalism gradually gave way to 'cooperative' federalism (Mathews 1977).

Expanded central activity during the Second World War and the reconstruction period, and the passage of the Uniform Tax Act in 1942, gave rise to a third phase of development that has been termed 'coercive' federalism (Mathews 1977: 8). Uniform income-tax legislation, upheld by the High Court, gave the Commonwealth a monopoly on income taxation. Although various revenue-sharing arrangements have operated since, financial power has remained very centralized. After 1942, the High Court returned briefly to a more limited interpretation of federal power. On the whole, however, the trend has been towards increased central power. The arbitration and conciliation power, the defence power, the external-affairs power, and the tax power have been interpreted generously (Sawer 1977a: 15–16). Since 1977, the corporations power and the external-affairs power have both been significantly extended.

TABLE 2
Revenues from own sources as a percentage of total government revenues by order of government, 1975 and 1985

	1975		1985	
	Federal	Provincial/ Local	Federal	Provincial/ Local
Australia	77.7	22.3	80.8	19.2
United States	55.8	44.2	56.3	43.7
West Germany	49.4	50.6	50.7	49.3
Canada	50.0	50.0	47.6	52.4
Switzerland	43.1	56.9	42.2	57.8

SOURCES: Government of Canada (1981: 37); OECD (1987: 204–32).
NOTE: Excludes contributions to social-security programs, i.e., programs that are organized separately from other activities of governments. Excludes revenue raised by supranational authorities. In practice, the only relevant institutions are those of the European Communities. To the extent that this table does not take into account the unconditional nature of some federal transfers to the provinces, for example, equalization payments, it understates the extent of Canadian financial decentralization.

The acceptance of Keynesian economics, and of a larger role for government generally, gave rise to vastly expanded Commonwealth activity by the Labor government in the post-war reconstruction period. Despite non-Labor's efforts to reverse some of these policies between 1949 and 1972, the centralization of financial power increased. There were indications that, under the 'new federalism' policy of the non-Labor government elected in 1975, there would be a return to a more cooperative federal style (Else-Mitchell 1975: 109–21) but, by 1982, it was apparent that the only changes had been in the direction of increased central control (Mathews 1983: 39–40). It is now widely accepted that the federal government has responsibility for managing the national economy. In carrying out this task, it largely determines tax rates and overall spending by both levels of government. In economic policy, the states are 'prepared to play second fiddle to the Commonwealth generally' (Solomon 1983: 76).

One illustration of the centralization of power in federations is the degree of revenue resources controlled by different levels of government. Table 2 shows the percentage of revenues by subsectors of government for the five major OECD federations.

Financial power is clearly far more centralized in Australia than in any of the other four nations. In contrast, only Switzerland was more decentralized than Canada in 1985. Table 2 also shows that, between 1975 and 1985, the trend towards financial centralization continued in Australia whereas further decentralization took place in Canada.

Thus, both the Canadian and Australian federations have altered radically in the course of their evolution. As Hodgins has summarized developments, 'by 1880 in Canada and by 1914 in Australia, the trend away from the intention of the Fathers was significant. It would, with interruptions, complications and contradictions continue. Today, Canada is one of the most decentralised operative federations in the world and Australia is one of the more centralised ones' (1978: 4).

Contrasting attitudes towards federalism appear to be both a reflection and a cause of 'the degree of federalness' in the two countries. Whereas Australians have argued for and against federalism in terms that reflect the ideas of 'orthodox' theories, Canadians have tended not to question the system as such but rather to examine the appropriateness or otherwise of various federal arrangements. Australian writers who have roundly condemned the system, using orthodox arguments, include Canaway (1930), Greenwood (1946), and Crisp (1949). As Sharman (1975) has noted, the debate between centralists and decentralists has changed little since the 1940s, although the centralist case has been propounded more fully and more frequently.

The federalism policies of the two major political parties are closely identified with the Australian debate on federalism. Since the early days of federation, the Australian Labor party has taken an anti-federalist stance, in the belief that the division of power prevented the possibility of controlling the economy and militated against the implementation of a social-democratic program. Non-Labor, in contrast, has always claimed to support federalism as a means of protecting society from the menace of Labor's collectivist policies, although, in the post-war period, Liberal–Country party governments presided over the centralization of economic and financial power (Starr 1977: 7–26; Wilenski 1983: 79–96).

Conflict between federalists and anti-federalists perhaps reached its height in the 1970s and is reflected in the two 'New Federalism' policies that emerged at the time. The Whitlam Labor government (1972–5) pursued a strongly centralist course, especially in areas of social policy. When it was returned to office in 1975, non-Labor stated that its objectives were to reverse the centralization of power and 'to return responsibility and revenue to those levels of government closest to the people' (Liberal Party of Australia 1978: 1). It soon became clear, however, that the real purpose of the exercise was not to return power to the states but rather to reduce

Commonwealth responsibility in some policy areas and to strengthen Commonwealth control over state finances (Sawer 1977c: 8; Cranston 1979: 136–42; Mathews 1983: 37–62; Solomon 1983: 75–6).

The federalism policies of the major Australian parties, then, are heavily interwoven with different views of the purpose of government. As one analyst has written of the two 'new federalisms,'

> their real goals, methods and philosophical justifications ... were markedly different and symbolized what has become the most emphatic perpetual distinction between the two sides in the Australian political contest. This distinction has deep ideological undertones relating directly to the parties' fundamental perceptions of the proper role of government. The Labor Party's position is perhaps best summarized by its platform planks calling for 'national planning of the economic, social and cultural development of Australia' ... The Liberal recognizes a 'right and obligation of the State to intervene' but only 'whenever such intervention can be clearly shown to be necessary.' (Starr 1977: 7–8)

The intensely ideological nature of the Australian debate contrasts strongly with the situation in Canada, where most writers have been concerned to analyse the evolution and operation of the federal system (see, for example, Lower and Scott 1958; Meekison 1977; Smiley 1980; Banting 1982, 1987). Controversy has tended to focus upon the appropriate balance of power between levels of government rather than on the merits and demerits of federalism as a system of government. As Stevenson (1979: 20) argues, 'most Canadians have found it so difficult to imagine alternatives to federalism that ... they have not considered it worthwhile to evaluate something that seems to be their inevitable fate. Since a unitary Canadian state has seemed beyond the realm of possibility, Canadian concepts of federalism have differed in many respects, but have resembled one another in taking federalism itself for granted.' In the division of constitutional responsibility for health policy there are also important differences between the two federations.

Constitutional Responsibility for Health

In both Canada and Australia, the power of the federal government in the health area was initially very limited. To the extent that government was to be involved at all, health-services provision in Canada was viewed as a local matter in 1867. Section 92 (7) of the BNA Act gives exclusive power to the provinces for 'the Establishment, Maintenance and Management of Hospitals, Asylums, Charities and Eleemosynary Institutions in and for the Province, other than Marine Hospitals.' The exclusive powers of the Dominion include 'militia, Military, and Naval Service and Defence' (Section 91 [7]), 'Indians and Lands reserved for the Indians' (Section 91 [7]) and 'Quarantine and the Establishment and Maintenance of Marine Hospitals' (Section 91 [11]). The constitutional authority of the Dominion was therefore restricted to the provision of health services for native people and members of the armed forces. In addition, a few public-health matters, such as the regulation of food and drug standards, became national functions.

In a major review of the federal balance of power in 1940, the Royal Commission on Dominion-Provincial Relations recommended that public and general health services should remain a provincial responsibility. Although the BNA Act, understandably, does not mention health insurance, the commission was of the view that any such scheme should be closely coordinated with other health services, especially those for low-income groups. It therefore recommended that the provinces be responsible for any health-insurance schemes that might be introduced. This location of legislative competence has persisted: the authority of the federal government is restricted to the conditions it is able to attach to its financial contributions towards provincial programs. In practice, these conditions are limited to the determination of a set of national standards in relation to the operation of the health-insurance system.

In Australia, responsibility for health services was originally one of the residual powers that remained with the states. Commonwealth involvement was restricted to matters of quarantine. As in many other policy areas, however, the federal government gradually extended its role. A Commonwealth department of health was established in 1921. After this time, the federal government began to assist the states with the provision of public-health services. In 1946, a constitutional amendment was enacted that gave the Commonwealth very wide concurrent powers in all aspects of health policy. Since the Second World War, the Commonwealth has dominated the policy-making process whereas, in Canada, the provinces have remained the senior level of government.

Federalism and Public-Policy Analysis[3]

Many writers besides students of federalism have attempted to explain the output of governments primarily in terms of the impact of a single variable. For example, King (1973) has argued that the pattern of American public policy is explained by distinctive ideas in that country about the appropriate role of government. Other writers, including Dye (1966), have argued that environmental factors, especially levels of economic development, are the most important determinants of policy. This approach has been challenged by Castles and McKinlay (1979a, 1979b) who argue that politics and, in particular, the strength of working-class movements and party ideology are vitally important. In a study of the development of selected social policies in Britain and Sweden, Heclo (1974: 301–4), choosing 'one group among all the separate political factors,' concludes that the bureaucracies in both countries played the most important and continuous role in policy formulation. Another factor identified as influencing the expansion of public expenditure is economic vulnerability in small, open economies with high levels of dependence on external trade (Cameron 1978; Banting 1990). Recently, Castles (1988) has advanced the argument that the closed nature of the economy is one of the main reasons for the underdevelopment of the Australian welfare state.

The variety of factors that have been found to influence what governments do has led some writers to stress the complexity, uncertainty, and diversity of policy determinants. Hawker, Smith, and Weller (1979: 22–3), for example, argue that 'public policy consists of continuing patterns of political and administrative activity that are shaped both by deliberate decisions and by the interplay of political and environmental forces. The sources of policy include strategic individuals in powerful organisations who attempt to shape policy in their own design, past patterns of policy, the political processes and structures through which policy proposals pass and the political and social environment in which relevant activity takes place.'

Similarly, Simeon (1976: 550) contends that 'policy emerges from the play of economic, social and political forces as manifested through institutions and processes.' He argues, therefore, that it is not enough to focus on one or two factors, such as the activities of 'proximate' policy makers or socio-economic conditions, in public-policy analysis. Moreover, he draws attention to the very difficult task of isolating the independent effect of institutions, arguing that 'institutional factors are so bound up with the other approaches that it seems impossible to weigh their overall impact on policy ... institutions themselves have no particular policy content; their effects lie in the way they interact with other social forces, and in the way they give advantages to some interests and disadvantages to others' (575).

In an attempt to overcome some of the shortcomings of policy studies that focus narrowly on one or two variables or on factors immediately surrounding certain decisions, Simeon (1976) developed a framework for the study of public policy. He suggests that several of the single perspectives taken by different analysts should be combined with a 'process' approach in policy research. The process approach, which examines the activities of proximate policy makers, is broadened to take into account other sets of influences, such as power, ideas, institutions, and the environment. Simeon further suggests that policy studies should be comparative and should be set in historical perspective. He acknowledges that the task for policy research that he outlines is 'a vast one,' fraught with many difficulties. However, as far as possible, a broad process approach set in historical and comparative perspectives such as that suggested by Simeon will be followed in the studies below.

A Note on Method

The task of comprehensive policy analysis can be simplified by selecting for study cases that have many characteristics in common. Such is particularly the case in the field of comparative politics, where analysts have devised what is called the 'most-similar systems' design. In studies based on this method, countries 'as similar as possible with respect to as many features as possible' are selected for examination. In this way, many potential variables are controlled for and 'the number of "experimental" variables ... is minimized' (Przeworski and Teune 1970: 32–3). Contrasting patterns of behaviour and policy outcomes can then be explained by differences between otherwise similar systems. Comparable cases 'offer particularly good opportunities for the application of the comparative method because they allow the establishment of relationships among a few variables while many other variables are controlled' (Lijphart 1971: 687).

Because of the many shared characteristics, Canada and Australia are therefore very suitable countries for comparative analysis. The design of this study, however, does not completely comply with the requirements of the 'most-similar systems' design. Ideally, the cases chosen, while being as alike as possible, should be different in respect to the main variable(s) being examined – in this instance, the impact of federal institutions. Strictly, a sound methodological approach would require that two (or more) similar countries, one a federal and the other a unitary system, be examined in order to identify the effects of the federal variable.[4] Despite this shortcoming, there is a great deal to be gained from comparing the two federations in question. First, the evidence can be scanned for instances of obstruction, deadlock, and the other predictions of orthodox theories. Second, the interaction of the impact of federal institutions with other policy determinants can be studied. Third, policy processes can be examined for common patterns or events in the two federations that may be attributable to divided power. If the findings are that the two systems operate quite differently from each other or over time, then the general validity of federal theories must be questioned. Finally, although Canada and Australia are both federations, they comply with the 'most-similar systems' design in their contrasting federal arrangements. Thus, the implications of different degrees of centralization and decentralization can be explored.

What this study cannot establish with confidence is that there is not something intrinsic to federalism operating in both countries that would only show up if comparison were made with unitary systems.[5] For example, it is possible, even without case-study evidence of delay and deadlock, that Canada and Australia lagged far behind unitary countries in health-policy development. This problem can be overcome to a large extent by cross-reference to developments in otherwise similar unitary systems. Thus, at various points in the analysis, British and New Zealand experience will be surveyed briefly.

Conclusion

It is in the context of very different institutional arrangements that the development of health policy in Canada and Australia must be examined and compared. If the proposition that fragmented power gives rise to limited government is accepted, then government in Canada should have been less interventionist than in Australia. If, by contrast, we accept the 'revisionist' arguments that many activist governments may contribute to policy expansion and government growth, then the reverse should be the case. In fact, at different times and in different ways, regional and central governments in both countries have actively promoted policy development, and, at the end of the 1980s, the Canadian and Australian health systems are remarkably similar. In the chapters that follow, the influences that have led to this outcome will be explored.

2

The Development of National Health
Insurance in Canada, 1900–70

After several unsuccessful provincial initiatives before the Second World War, the governments of Canada formulated and implemented a comprehensive system of national health insurance in the post-war period. As mentioned in the introduction, health is an area fraught with difficulties for public-policy makers. Not only are powerful interest groups, particularly the medical profession, opposed to most government intervention but the assumption of responsibility for health insurance involves government in large and frequently unpredictable budgetary outlays. Even the design of an efficient administrative system presents a major challenge. Yet the various Canadian governments between them overcame these difficulties. Medicare, as the health-insurance system came to be known, is one of the country's most popular public programs. This chapter traces the development of national health insurance in Canada from the time of the first initiatives in the western provinces in the early years of the century until its full implementation as a national system in the late 1960s.

Provincial Policy Initiatives Prior to the Second World War

Before the Second World War, federal-government involvement in Canadian health policy was minimal (Cassidy 1945: 8). Except for psychiatric hospitals, interest in the direct government provision of hospital and medical services and health insurance was confined to western Canada. However, governments in all provinces, as in Britain and other comparable countries, became involved in the provision of public-health services in the last quarter of the nineteenth century (Hastings and Mosely 1980: 148–51; Cassidy 1945: 33–143, 452–3). In the 1960s, the report of the Royal Commission on Health Services (hereafter referred to as the Hall Report) found that Canadian mortality and morbidity rates were comparable with those of countries with similar levels of socio-economic development, except among Indian and Inuit people in the isolated North (Hall Report 1964: 149–54, 225–6). The development and efficacy of public-health services in Canada appear to have paralleled those in other countries.

In the eastern and central provinces, however, there was almost no government involvement in the provision of general hospital facilities or medical services, although some services for the poor were provided through public-health boards. The royal commission of 1964 suggested that higher population density and greater philanthropic support for hospitals from large private fortunes made the private provision of health services more viable and reduced the need for government intervention (Hall Report 1964: 383). In 1935, Newfoundland, which did not enter confederation until after the Second World War, introduced the Cottage Hospital and Medical Care plan, which provided an extensive range of services. Ontario came to an agreement with the medical profession in 1935 under which a fund was established to provide a small subsidy for medical services for welfare recipients. The fund was administered by the medical profession (Brown 1983: 35). Otherwise, the provision of health services was a private matter in eastern and central Canada.

By contrast, in the west there were a number of attempts to establish health-insurance schemes prior to the Second World War. There were also government-sponsored schemes for the direct provision of hospital and medical services, although, as we shall see in the next chapter, government involvement in service provision was far less extensive in Canada than in the Australian states at the time. The initiatives in western Canada had their basis in the strong cooperative movement that had emerged in the prairie provinces by the turn of the century. Despite, or perhaps because of, the economic devastation of the region during the depression, the cooperative movement gained momentum throughout the 1930s. Credit unions, life-insurance plans, the manufacture of farm equipment, an oil refinery, and recreational programs[1] were established on a collective basis (Macpherson 1979: 3–21).

In this distinctive environment, a new political party, the Cooperative Commonwealth Federation (CCF), was formed in 1932. The founders of the party believed that the social and economic relations of society could be transformed by democratic means. Among the wide range of policies developed by the party was a proposal for extensive government intervention in the health sector. The manifesto of the party declared that 'health services should be made as freely available as are educational services today. But under a system which is still mainly one of private enterprise, the costs of proper medical care, such as the wealthier members of society can easily afford, are at present prohibitive for great masses of people' (Regina Manifesto July 1933: 6).

In the course of the next few decades, the CCF and its successor, the New Democratic Party (NDP), had a profound influence on the development of Canadian health policy. The policies announced in 1933 were not, however, a radical break with the past but were rather an expansion of previous initiatives in the western provinces.

Early Initiatives in Service Provision and Attempts to Introduce Insurance

In 1909, the Saskatchewan government passed legislation enabling the municipalities to provide hospital facilities and services by means of local taxation, a system that steadily expanded (Taylor 1978: 72). The Municipal Doctor Scheme was introduced in the Saskatchewan municipality of Sarnia in 1914. Under this scheme, municipalities contracted with doctors to provide medical services, which usually included general services, maternity care, and minor surgery. Doctors were paid an annual retainer. By 1948, the system operated in 107 municipalities, 14 towns, and 59 villages in Saskatchewan and had spread to the neighbouring provinces of Alberta and Manitoba, although on a more limited scale (Hall Report 1964: 385).

Besides these innovations in service provision, there was extensive interest in all four western provinces in the development of public-health insurance. In Saskatchewan, a small group of people formed what later became the State Hospital and Medical League in Prince Albert in 1933. According to one of the founders, few people had money to pay for medical services, and the local doctor was on relief.[2] The league gathered information about services in other countries and pressured both provincial and federal governments for the introduction of health insurance. Both were unsympathetic but, under pressure from the CCF, the provincial Liberal government introduced health-insurance legislation in 1944 just before it lost office to the CCF (Taylor 1978: 74–7).

Health insurance became a political issue in Alberta in the late 1920s.

After two inquiries, legislation for a comprehensive scheme was passed in April 1935. Political events intervened, however, and the act was never promulgated. A special select committee was established to study the Manitoba health system in 1931. The committee recommended a mixed scheme of insurance and directly provided services, including expansion of the Municipal Doctor Scheme and the municipal hospital system. It suggested that a commission be established to formulate detailed proposals. The commission was not established, but the Municipal Doctor Scheme was later expanded (Hall Report 1964: 394–7; Taylor 1949: 50–3; Gelber 1980: 161).

Public demand for health insurance was strong in British Columbia. The issue was raised many times in the legislature from 1919 onwards but the medical profession strongly opposed government intervention. A royal commission was eventually established, and its 1932 report recommended a scheme very similar to the British system: compulsory insurance for those earning less than $200 per month. The medical profession vehemently opposed the proposal, arguing that the income limit was too high and that people who could afford to pay private fees would be included. The doctors were supported by the Manufacturer's Association, which was against the imposition of employer contributions.

In the November 1933 election, the Conservative government was resoundingly defeated. The Liberal party was elected, and the new CCF won 7 seats and 31.1 per cent of the vote (Simerl 1982: 690–3). After lengthy negotiations with the profession, the insurance proposals were redrafted, with the help of a member of the Canadian Medical Association (CMA) who had been nominated by the local branch of the profession. Most of the recommendations of the doctors and the manufacturers were adopted, but both groups remained strongly opposed to the plan. Two weeks before health insurance was due to come into operation in 1937, the government announced that the scheme would be postponed until after the forthcoming election. Although returned to power, the government made no further attempt to proceed with the policy (Taylor 1949: 15–38).

Despite the failure to establish a health-insurance plan in any of the four provinces, these initiatives were not without consequence. There was strong public support for government action, particularly in British Columbia and Saskatchewan. The various inquiries and commissions had gathered and disseminated a great deal of information, and wide public debate had taken place. Thus a foundation was provided for the policies that were introduced after the Second World War. The climate of public opinion in the west and the challenge presented by the increasing electoral success of the CCF in both federal and provincial jurisdictions were among the reasons that the federal government undertook a review of the whole question of social policy during the Second World War.

Health Policy and the Federal Government

As discussed in chapter 1, the constitutional power of the federal government in health policy is very limited. Prior to the 1960s, however, the use of the conditional grant was widely accepted, and such grants were frequently employed by the federal government to influence policies outside its jurisdiction, particularly in education and pensions. In contrast, there had only been one small cost-shared health program prior to the 1940s (Brown 1984: 11–14; Bryden 1974: 61–101). Throughout the depression, the federal government maintained that relief for medical care was a provincial responsibility, although it had given assistance for other forms of relief (Taylor 1949: 65–6). Health, it seems, was an area that successive federal governments were content to leave to the provinces.

As in most Western countries, social policy became a prominent issue in Canada during the Second World War. The federal Liberal government, however, was slow to respond, lagging behind both the CCF and the Conservative party in developing new policies. As the war dragged on, the government's policy of winning the war before making plans for the post-war period came under criticism. The Wartime Information Board reported that people dreaded the coming of peace and feared a return to the conditions of the 1930s. They wanted a different society once the war was over and wanted to know what the government intended to do (Granatstein 1975: 251).

The climate of opinion was reflected in growing support for the CCF, which, in addition to successes in the western provinces, established itself federally in the early 1940s. The Conservative party responded quickly to the increasing support for the left. It devised a range of social-policy reforms, renamed itself the Progressive Conservative party, and 'set out to defeat the CCF and its socialism and Mackenzie King and his policies of delay and evasion' (Granatstein 1975: 252). The government, however, was not committed. Many members of Cabinet either were not interested in social-policy reform or were actively hostile. The prime minister, Mackenzie King, complained that 'the mind of the Cabinet ... does not grasp the significance of the Beveridge Report [*Report of the Interdepartmental Committee on Social Insurance and Allied Services, United Kingdom, 1942*] ... the effect the war is having on some members of the government [is] to make them so reactionary as to cause the party generally to lose ground right along to the CCF' (quoted in Granatstein 1975: 262). However, although the prime minister often spoke in support of social-policy reform, his position appears to have been ambivalent (Granatstein 1975: 263–81).

There was nevertheless one member of Cabinet, Ian Mackenzie, from British Columbia, who was firmly committed to the introduction of new social policies, including national health insurance. He became Minister for Pensions and Health in 1939, and his efforts were largely responsible for making health insurance an important issue within the federal government (Granatstein 1975: 254). He urged the prime minister to introduce health insurance as a wartime measure and was instrumental in having established the Interdepartmental Advisory Committee on Health Insurance (the Heagerty Committee) and the Advisory Committee on Reconstruction. Although the power of the Committee on Reconstruction was undermined by the Economic Advisory Committee, it continued with its work and produced the Marsh Report in 1943. This report was 'hailed immediately throughout the country as the Canadian Beveridge Plan' (Cassidy 1945: 1).

Meanwhile, Mackenzie had discussed health insurance with the Dominion Council of Health, a body of provincial health officials and representatives of the medical profession, farm, labour, and women's groups. There was wide support for health insurance, and the minister suggested that the provinces formulate detailed plans for presentation to the federal government.

The Heagerty Committee, which had worked very closely with a special committee of the CMA, produced a comprehensive report at the end of 1942. It provided an extensive review of health services in Canada and in other countries and recommended a universal system of compulsory health insurance for Canada. The federal government should offer to share the costs with the provinces, it suggested, by means of a grant-in-aid (Taylor 1978: 17–18; Naylor 1986: 102–4).

Draft legislation was prepared by Mackenzie's department and presented to Cabinet in January 1943. The matter was referred to the Economic Advisory Committee, which objected strenuously to the proposals. Mackenzie wrote to the prime minister, threatening to resign. The proposals were brought to Cabinet again later in the month but were again opposed by the Department of Finance. As a compromise, the House of Commons Special Committee on Social Security was established to study the whole question of social insurance, a fall-back position suggested by Mackenzie.

In the course of its deliberations, the Special Committee heard representations from a wide range of groups, including the CMA and Sir William Beveridge. Its first report was presented in July 1943, and, while it endorsed the principles of the draft legislation, it reserved judgment on the financial estimates. After consideration by yet another committee, the legislation was redrafted and given approval by the House of Commons Special Committee (Taylor 1978: 20–38).

By the end of 1943, however, electoral considerations had become Cabinet's top priority. The Liberals had been decisively defeated in four federal by-elections in 1943. An opinion poll showed that there was slightly more support for the CCF than for either of the two main parties. Cabinet was still divided on the question of appropriate reconstruction policies. The Minister of Finance was strongly opposed to any measure that would increase federal expenditures, unless the federal government could retain control of the major tax-revenue fields that had been 'rented' to it by the provinces as a wartime measure. Despite this division, it was announced in January 1944 that a wide range of social-policy initiatives would be taken (Granatstein 1975: 272–6).

The federal government then began work on the preparation of an agenda for a dominion–provincial conference, which had to be held because the tax-rental agreements were due to expire one year after the end of hostilities. In this context, a number of possible social-policy initiatives were discussed. Finally, in July 1944, Cabinet decided that health insurance would be shelved for the time being, but that family allowances would be introduced. At the same time, Mackenzie was removed from his portfolio, and Brooke Claxton, who later openly opposed health insurance, became minister for the reorganized Department of Health and Welfare (Taylor 1978: 39–45, 220).

In 1945, all parties campaigned on platforms that included proposals for health insurance. Opinion polls showed that 80 per cent of people supported a national plan. The Liberal government was returned with a narrow majority, but both the Progressive Conservatives and the CCF made significant gains (Taylor 1978: 43–8). A limited health-insurance scheme was part of the federal package put to the Dominion–Provincial Conference in 1945. The federal government offered to meet 60 per cent of estimated costs, but the estimates were low and would have resulted in a federal share of only about 40 per cent (Hall Report 1964: 403–4). It also offered to assume full responsibility for old-age pensions and unemployment assistance. In return, the provinces were asked to vacate the fields of income and corporation taxes, succession duties, and several minor taxation fields. Thus, federal financial assistance for health insurance was to be achieved at the cost of conceding to the federal Department of Finance most of its long-term taxation aims.

The Failure to Reach Agreement

After three days of deliberation, the conference adjourned to allow the provinces to consider the proposals. By January 1946, it seemed that there was a general willingness to vacate the fields of income and corporation taxes, but both Ontario and Quebec wanted to retain control of succession duties. The prime minister sympathized with this view and was of the opinion that the level of government that spends money should be responsible for raising the necessary taxes (Taylor 1978: 62).

When the conference reconvened in April 1946, the three prairie provinces had agreed to accept the federal offer as it stood. All the provinces were willing to vacate the personal- and corporation-tax fields, and six, possibly seven, were willing to give up succession duties. However, the view of the federal Department of Finance prevailed, and no compromises were made on the original offer. The conference ended without agreement, and the health-insurance proposals were set aside indefinitely (Taylor 1978: 61–5).

The failure of the conference appears at first sight to be an example of federal obstacles to policy development. However, closer inspection casts doubt on such a conclusion. Clearly there was little support in Cabinet for health insurance. Without the efforts of Mackenzie and the growing electoral support for the CCF it seems unlikely that the issue would have been on the conference agenda at all.

In view of the radical nature of the revenue-sharing proposals and the uncompromising stance of the federal government, it is not surprising that the conference failed. Indeed, it is more surprising that agreement was nearly reached. The proportion of taxation revenue that gave rise to the deadlock was less than 5 per cent and was raised in seven different tax fields, so that a number of compromise solutions were possible.

The primary concern of Cabinet was management of the post-war economy to prevent a return to depression conditions. The Minister of Finance was a central actor and opposed all social-policy proposals (Granatstein 1975: 253–84). If Canada's had been a unitary system, it seems most unlikely that Cabinet would have approved of any measure not central to its economic objectives in 1946, especially since another election was not required for four years.

Health insurance was not taken up at the federal level again until 1955, and then only reluctantly in the face of strong provincial and electoral pressure. In the meantime, however, the western provinces proceeded with the development and implementation of their own health schemes. It is at least arguable that policy development was advanced as quickly by the successful introduction of comprehensive measures at the provincial level, which were later taken up nationally, as it would have been if the limited federal proposals had been implemented.

The Saskatchewan Hospital Services Plan

At the 1944 provincial election, the CCF was elected to government and won 47 of the 52 seats in the Saskatchewan legislature. The new premier, ex–Baptist minister Tommy Douglas, was strongly committed to the development of comprehensive health services, which would be universally available without consideration of ability to pay. There were considerable obstacles to the implementation of such a program, however. In the first place, the province was heavily in debt. Second, there was no health-insurance scheme in operation anywhere in North America from which to learn (McLeod 1971: 82–5). The province's difficult financial situation was exacerbated in 1944 when federal Finance minister J.L. Ilsley called in a loan of $16.5 million (Shackleton 1975: 164–5). Nevertheless, planning for health reforms went ahead. The Health Services Planning Commission (HSPC) was established, and a wide range of services, including free treatment for cancer, psychiatric, and pensioner and other low-income patients, were established (McLeod 1971: 87; Shackleton 1975: 232; Taylor 1978: 102).

Apart from financial constraints, the government was faced with physician opposition to many of its proposals (Shackleton 1975: 164–5). Regionalization, a well-established provincial tradition, accorded with the government's policy of decentralized, democratic control. The HSPC saw this as a means of providing services to undersupplied areas. The profession opposed locally elected health boards, which it could not control, and the regionalization of services, which would reduce the number of patients referred to the two major cities where most specialists were located. The Saskatchewan College of Physicians and Surgeons feared that its own power would be reduced because regional medical societies would negotiate separately with regional boards (Taylor 1978: 245).

The college was adamant that health insurance should be administered by 'a non-political independent commission,' and it vehemently opposed the expansion of the Municipal Doctor Scheme under which physicians were paid by salary. It was clear that only a fee-for-service system of remuneration would be acceptable. The government consequently modified its proposals. It agreed to the establishment of an independent commission. The question of medical services was set aside, partly because of the profession's objections and partly for financial reasons. A scheme for hospital insurance was given priority. The HSPC did succeed in having two health regions established, despite the college's attempts to persuade local medical societies not to cooperate (Taylor 1978: 245–51). In the Swift Current region, a full system of hospital and medical insurance was introduced, although existing salaried practice was replaced by fee-for-service (Brown 1983: 37). The project was successful and enjoyed the support of the community. It was later to influence the Royal Commission on Health Services in the early 1960s. Mr Justice Hall, chairman, reported that the scheme had been one of the most valuable sources of information available to the commission (Shackleton 1975: 232–3). Swift Current created a 'demonstration effect' and was a prototype of the national plan introduced in the late 1960s. The abolition of salaried practice was thus a very important victory for the profession and paved the way for a national medical-insurance system in which doctors are paid on a fee-for-service basis.

In contrast, hospital insurance was relatively uncontroversial. The planning of the scheme involved many groups and conflict was reduced to a minimum. The Saskatchewan Hospitals Services Plan began operation on 1 January 1947. Of the 'demonstration effect' of the scheme, the royal commission of 1964 said 'the Saskatchewan Hospital Plan served as a testing ground for the solution of many problems associated with universal coverage and administration by a government body. In 1948, when British Columbia and Alberta were considering the introduction of their programmes and again from 1956 to 1960, when other provinces were preparing to accept the terms of the National Hospital Insurance Act, all the provinces sent delegations to study the Saskatchewan organization and procedures' (Hall Report 1964: 408).

Following the Saskatchewan example, hospital insurance was introduced in British Columbia in 1948 and in Alberta, on a more limited basis, in 1950. Whereas the Saskatchewan and British Columbia plans were centrally administered, the Alberta plan involved 50–50 cost sharing between the provincial government and the municipalities. Some services were not covered, and not all municipalities developed insurance plans. Nevertheless, by 1954 three-quarters of Alberta hospital patients were insured under the program (Hall Report 1964: 409–10).

It was clearly in the interests of the three western provinces that the federal government renew its 1945 cost-sharing offer. However, at the 1950 Federal–Provincial Conference, Prime Minister St Laurent made it clear that the 1945 proposals were no longer considered an appropriate course of action. Concern about the financial burden that would be created by an expansion of social services was still the overriding consideration (Taylor 1978: 165–85).[3] However, public demand for a comprehensive health-insurance scheme had not abated. In 1949, as in 1944, 80 per cent of the population approved of a scheme under which the costs of health care would be met on a prepaid basis (Taylor 1978: 166).

The National Hospital Insurance Plan

In 1955, the Conservative premier of Ontario suggested that a joint national health-insurance program should be put on the agenda for the next federal–provincial conference. It was only after Health and Welfare minister Paul Martin, who was as committed to health insurance as was Ian Mackenzie, threatened to resign, that the prime minister agreed to the inclusion of the item. At the conference a committee was established to study national health insurance.

An intense political struggle took place over the next two years between the federal government, which continued to try to delay action, and Premier Frost, who was determined not to proceed without federal financial assistance (Taylor 1978: 104–238). Under pressure from the provinces and the CCF, and with strong public support for health insurance, the federal government made an offer in January 1956, but the terms and conditions were not conducive to ready acceptance (*Globe and Mail* 25 January 1956: 1). Negotiations and political games continued between Ottawa and Ontario throughout 1956 and 1957, but the political costs of delay began to mount, especially for the federal government. In 1957, an election year, the Conservative opposition in Ottawa supported the proposals.

In the end, both governments took action. The necessary legislation was passed in Ontario in March 1957, and in Ottawa in April. The reaction in the House of Commons appears to reflect intense support for the scheme. As one newspaper reported the scene: 'to tumultuous applause, the Commons tonight gave third and final reading to the proposed national hospital insurance plan. Cheers echoed through the Chamber as the House voted 165–0 for the scheme ... Stanley Knowles (CCF), long-time battler for a hospital insurance scheme, requested the formal division. Prolonged desk-thumping broke out as Prime Minister St Laurent rose to vote. More applause greeted Health Minister Martin, Opposition Leader Diefenbaker, Mr Knowles and Reverend E.G. Hansell (S.C. McLeod) as they voted in their turn' (*Globe and Mail* 11 April 1959: 1). If members were playing to the electorate, very wide support for the scheme must have been thought to exist.

One by one, federal-provincial agreements were signed, a process that was facilitated by the defeat of the federal government later in the year. Prime Minister Diefenbaker agreed to begin cost-sharing with those provinces already operating eligible plans rather than wait for five provinces with a majority of the population to come into the scheme.[4] Cost-sharing began with the four western provinces and Newfoundland on 1 July 1958. Ontario and Nova Scotia had implemented plans by 1 January 1959, and Prince Edward Island and New Brunswick followed later in the year. Quebec, traditionally opposed to federal intervention in areas of provincial jurisdiction, entered the scheme on 1 January 1961 in the wake of the Lesage Liberal victory that marked the onset of what became known as that province's Quiet Revolution (Brown 1983: 41). Once in operation, the scheme worked well. The royal commission reported that 'the programme appears to us to be a sound blend of federal financial support and respect for provincial responsibility. In fact, it goes beyond that for in its administration it utilises a number of joint Federal–Provincial committees and working parties. It is a remarkably successful example of what has long been termed "cooperative federalism"' (Hall Report 1964: 413).

Federalism, then, does not always involve conflict and political difficulties. Once the system was established, a high level of consensus emerged. As we will see in later chapters, the chances of conflict occurring are increased if powerful interest groups are opposed to a policy. In this case, although the medical profession did not welcome hospital insurance, it was not strongly opposed.

By the end of the 1950s, a system of medical insurance was the one unfulfilled part of the Saskatchewan government's 1944 plan to provide universal access to a comprehensive range of health services. The receipt of federal assistance for hospital expenditures made the introduction of medical insurance financially easier. However, before medical insurance could be introduced in Saskatchewan, the government had to face a long and bitter confrontation with the College of Physicians and Surgeons.

The Introduction of Medical Insurance in Saskatchewan

Although the Canadian medical profession wished to limit government intervention in health policy in order to preserve its economic and clinical autonomy as far as possible, it was aware of the potential benefits of schemes that would enable low-income earners to pay fees. The steep increase in the numbers of people who could not afford to pay and the consequent decline in medical incomes during the depression led to a general acceptance of health insurance for low-income groups and even some support for universal insurance and for capitation payments for general practitioners (Naylor 1986: 58–134; Brown 1983: 35–6). Thus, the CMA worked closely with the Heagerty Committee during the Second World War, when political considerations indicated that some form of health insurance was inevitable. Naylor (1986: 247) describes the wartime CMA approach as 'a loss-minimizing strategy.'

Support for government insurance was far from unanimous, however, and alternative arrangements were explored, which, it was hoped, would obviate the need for a public scheme. From the late 1930s onwards, physicians began to foster the development of voluntary insurance. Brown argues that the profession would have preferred to leave insurance to commercial companies but that 'it realised that good private plans were necessary to fight the introduction of socialised medicine. Since good private plans implied some control over medical practitioner pricing, the medical organisations were forced to become involved' (1983: 39).

The schemes that were subsequently developed were known as 'service' plans or 'participating doctor schemes.' Doctors who agreed to participate undertook not to charge patients but to send their bills directly to the plan. In most cases, the patient was not involved in paying a fee. This system differs substantially from a reimbursement scheme, where the patient pays the doctor and then seeks reimbursement from a fund. A reimbursement plan can operate regardless of the fee charged by the doctor. Patients are reimbursed by the amount of a stipulated benefit and meet any difference between the benefit and the fee themselves. Under the service contract, however, it is necessary for physician fees to be controlled, since premium levels can be calculated only on the basis of a known fee.

The advent of more prosperous economic conditions after the Second World War saw organized Canadian medicine swing 'sharply right' (Naylor 1986: 134). The CMA issued a policy statement in 1949 that proposed that government involvement be reduced to a minimum: instead of publicly administered insurance for low-income earners, the policy was that these people should be subsidized by governments to enrol in private plans administered and controlled by the profession (CMA *Journal*, 60 [February 1949]: 186; Naylor 1986: 152–8). Hospital insurance did not alter the way doctors were paid and was therefore introduced without serious opposition, but medical insurance would involve negotiations with governments over fee levels and modes of remuneration. Throughout the 1950s, private insurance was expanded, and, in 1960, doctor-sponsored plans and commercial plans were amalgamated in an attempt to provide national coverage and to form a common front against government (Taylor 1978: 335–8). Thus by the time Premier Douglas announced the decision to introduce a system of 'Prepaid Medical Care' in 1959, the medical profession 'had anticipated and was in no mood to accept government intrusion into its markets' (Brown 1983: 42).

The Saskatchewan profession was particularly well placed to resist government initiatives. In the first place, it was organized in a unique way. The voluntary Saskatchewan Medical Association had been amalgamated with the College of Physicians and Surgeons in 1936. The college was thus both the regulating and licensing body of the profession and its political arm. The annual licensing fee included membership in the association and was universal and compulsory, which prompted commentators to classify the college as a 'private government' (McLeod 1971: 89; Taylor 1978: 264–5) or as 'a state within a state' (*Montreal Star* 5 July 1962). Although it was clear that the college did not represent the views of the majority of municipal doctors, the government had been aware since 1947 that it would be politically difficult to try to break its monopolistic power (McLeod 1971: 89). Second, the province was short of doctors and has a harsh climate. The warning that doctors would leave the province thus carried considerable weight. Policy makers realized that any scheme would require the profession's cooperation in order to be successful. Thus, the government's preferred option of a decentralized, democratically controlled alternative delivery system, through which, it was hoped, services could be located in undersupplied areas, was abandoned. Even though major concessions had been made there were still problems in designing an acceptable system because the college insisted that there was no need for a government scheme at all. However, in April 1959, an interdepartmental committee was established to begin work on a medical-insurance scheme. The committee recommended that a representative public planning committee be established. The college at first refused to participate but eventually agreed to nominate representatives in return for changes in the committee's membership and an expansion of the agenda, a strategy designed to achieve delay (Taylor 1978: 270–81).

The provincial election of 1960 was virtually transformed into a referendum on the proposed scheme, which had become known as 'Medicare.' The college waged a large publicity campaign, financed by a $100 levy on members and a donation of $35,000 from the CMA. It was supported by the Liberal party, the pharmaceutical and dental associations, and the Chamber of Commerce. The CCF government was returned with a large majority of seats but did not win a majority of votes in the four-party contest. Although the CMA accepted the result, the Saskatchewan college did not.

Nevertheless the government decided to proceed. The Saskatchewan Medical Insurance Act of 1961 provided for a system of universal, compulsory insurance for the services of physicians and surgeons in home, office, or hospital. Initially, the college refused to recognize the act. However, after a number of invitations, meetings were held with the minister in March and April 1962. In an effort to gain cooperation, the government made a major concession. The legislation had provided that physicians would direct-bill the insurance commission according to an official fee schedule, in the manner that operated in the profession-sponsored plans. The government now conceded that doctors could present their bills directly to the patient at whatever fee they chose and that patients could then claim reimbursement from the commission. The offer was flatly rejected. The profession continued to demand that the government restrict its activities to the subsidization of private insurance premiums for low-income earners (Taylor 1978: 294–5).

The struggle that followed was bitter and created deep divisions in the community. When Medicare began operation on 1 July 1962, most of the province's doctors withdrew all but emergency services, and some left the province. Groups had formed to support both sides. A Keep Our Doctor's Committee (KODC) had been organized with the backing of the Liberal party and the American Medical Association. Meetings and rallies were held all over the province. According to Lord Taylor, the British doctor who served as a mediator between the government and the college, 'many of those who opposed Medicare saw in this struggle an opportunity to bring down the CCF government, at a time when the dynamic leadership of Tommy Douglas had just been removed' (quoted in CMA Journal 110 [6 April 1974]: 833). The prospect that doctors would leave the province also appears to have been a powerful factor in shaping people's opinions (CMA Journal 37 [27 October 1962]). At the same time, the Saskatchewan

Citizens for Medicare campaigned actively, and community health-service associations were formed in many areas for the purpose of providing clinics for those doctors who wished to work on a salaried basis. Long after the dispute was settled many doctors remained vehemently opposed to these clinics, three of which were still in operation in 1985.[5]

As the strike continued there were indications that 'the tide of pro-doctor opinion had begun to ebb' (Taylor 1978: 315). In the meantime, the government had been attempting to find a negotiator who would be acceptable to the profession. Lord Steven Taylor, physician, and former adviser to the British Labour Party, was invited to the province. After eight days of mediation, the 'Saskatoon Agreement' was reached and signed. Doctors returned to work on 23 July 1962, and a much modified Medicare began operation.[6]

Yet, as one observer has argued, 'it is possible to win the battle and lose the war.' The scheme was a far cry from the decentralized system originally envisaged by the government (McLeod 1971: 90). In addition, the government had 'backed down on its proposal to become a bargaining unit on behalf of patients.' Doctors had gained the right not to participate in the plan, a practice known as 'opting-out,' and had retained 'all the pricing powers that they had had in pre-medicare days' (Brown 1983: 43).

Nevertheless, the CCF government had managed to introduce a medical-insurance plan that eliminated the financial barriers restricting access to health services. If the electoral success of the CCF, which had been in power since 1944, can be used as a measure, then support for social-democratic policies was stronger in Saskatchewan than anywhere else in Canada. As a countervailing force to the power of the medical profession, this support was necessary to sustain the government through the two-year confrontation. It is most unlikely that any other government in Canada, where public support was weaker, could have succeeded in introducing Medicare.

The federal system, then, allowed both hospital- and medical-insurance plans to be introduced in a single province. Medicare proved to be both popular and administratively straightforward, and the success of the scheme undermined the medical profession's claims that patients' interests would be jeopardized in a variety of ways. In fact, within a short time, the scheme was accepted by the vast majority of Saskatchewan doctors. After fighting so hard for the right to 'opt out' of the plan, 95.8 per cent of doctors were sending their bills directly to the insurance commission by 1967, following the practice in the profession-sponsored plans

(Scotton and Deeble 1968: 12). As with hospital insurance, Medicare did not remain a uniquely Saskatchewan program. Within a decade, the scheme had been implemented on a national basis.

The National Medicare Program

While the CCF government in Saskatchewan was occupied with Medicare, two important developments took place that were instrumental in extending the program to the rest of the country. First, the federal Liberal party in opposition underwent a transformation. The old leadership was replaced. Under the new leader, Lester Pearson, the party platform was revised. A range of social policies were formulated, including a proposal for 'a medical care plan for all Canadians, established in cooperation with the provinces.' Second, the Royal Commission on Health Services had been appointed. The CMA, alarmed by developments in Saskatchewan, had approached Prime Minister Diefenbaker and requested an inquiry into health needs and health insurance. The move was an attempt to forestall the implementation of Medicare in Saskatchewan. It was hoped that the government would be forced to postpone action until the findings of the inquiry became available (Brown 1983: 44).

Under the chairmanship of Mr Justice Hall, the commission undertook a wide-ranging study of Canadian and international health services and presented its two-volume report in 1964. The recommendations in relation to health insurance were a bitter blow to the medical profession. The commission found that 'after more than 25 years of endeavour on the part of voluntary and commercial insurance companies, only slightly more than one-half of the population of Canada has any degree of voluntary insurance protection and this for medical services alone. Of these, the coverage held by nearly 3 million is wholly inadequate' (Hall Report, vol. 1 [1964]: 743).

As frequently happens in health policy, experience in one country influences policy development in another. The commission had studied the Australian voluntary health-insurance system and found that, after eleven years of operation, only 80 per cent of the population had insurance cover despite extensive government subsidization of the scheme (Hall Report, vol. 1 [1964]: 744). The heavy administrative costs of the Australian scheme were noted, and it was estimated that it would cost an additional $183 million per annum 'just to have physician's services alone administered by the health insurance industry' (vol. 1 [1964]: 744–5). Of the CMA proposal that government subsidies should be available to enable low-income earners to meet the costs of premiums, the commission said that 'the number of individuals who would require subsidy to meet total health services costs is so large that no government could impose the means test procedure on so many citizens or would be justified in establishing a system requiring so much unnecessary administration' (vol. 1 [1964]: 743). On the basis of its findings and determinations the commission concluded that 'the best solution for Canada is the establishment of a comprehensive, universal Health Services Programme ... Canada requires the establishment of health insurance funds, provincially administered, contributed to by the Federal Government from general revenue and by provincial governments as they may determine, structured along similar lines to the Hospital Insurance Programme' (vol. 1 [1964]: 743). The scheme was identical in principle to that operating in Saskatchewan. The medical profession and the insurance industry responded with outrage. In Taylor's view, the profession believed that its 'supplement, don't supplant' approach was so sound that no reasonable commission could fail to endorse it (1980: 188).

The Liberal party was returned to power in 1963 but failed to gain a majority of seats. On matters of social-policy reform it could count on support from the NDP, successor to the CCF, now led at the federal level by the ex-premier of Saskatchewan, Tommy Douglas. In line with the new social-policy approach and following the recommendations of the royal commission, Prime Minister Pearson called a federal-provincial conference in 1965 to discuss proposals for a national medical-insurance scheme. Because opposition had developed to the principle of cost-shared programs in Ontario and Quebec, conditions were kept to a minimum. Four principles were suggested: that the program should cover a comprehensive range of medical services; that it should be universal, covering all residents; that benefits should be portable between provinces; that the plan should be administered by a public agency (Taylor 1978: 364–5).[7]

Provincial responses were varied, but the only outright opposition came from the premier of Quebec, who announced his intention to establish his own plan. Health minister J. Donovan Ross of Alberta opposed the exclusion of commercial for-profit insurance carriers. Ontario wanted a major reallocation of revenue between levels of government before proceeding and wanted reimbursement of actual rather than national per-capita costs (*Report of the Parliamentary Task Force on Federal-Provincial Fiscal Arrangements* [Breau Report] 1981: 53).

Despite the objections of the two largest provinces, the medical profession, and the insurance industry, Cabinet decided to proceed. The prime minister, several senior ministers, and key segments of the Liberal party were committed to the policy as 'a vital piece of social legislation' (Weller 1974: 93). The NDP was effective in promoting the issue, especially in the House of Commons. Legislation was introduced in 1966 but, because of time constraints, had not been passed when the House rose for the summer recess. Thus, the forces of opposition were given an opportunity to mobilize, and a 'last-ditch offensive' was launched. The campaign focused on a regular meeting of provincial premiers that was held in August. The federal proposals were heavily criticized (Taylor 1978: 369). The most effective opposition, however, came not from the provinces or from interest groups but, as in the 1940s, from the Minister of Finance, at this time, Mitchell Sharp. He began to argue publicly that caution should be exercised in relation to the introduction of new social programs. The effects of such programs on the economy and on the rate of inflation should be considered, he suggested, and he openly cast doubt on the future of the Medicare proposals (*Globe and Mail* 8 September 1966: 1). In September, in his capacity as deputy prime minister while Mr Pearson was overseas, Mr Sharp announced in the House of Commons that the introduction of the scheme would be postponed. Several ministers spoke in public against the decision and Health minister Allan MacEachen considered resigning. The resulting furore within the Liberal party is said to have been matched only by the jubilation of the opponents of Medicare (Taylor 1978: 371).

On his return, the prime minister supported the Finance minister, and caucus members were forced to accept the postponement. At a Liberal convention held in October, the party, too, accepted the decision, but only on the condition that the delay would be for a maximum period of one year (Taylor 1978: 372).

The Medical Care Act was passed in the House of Commons in December 1966 by a vote of 172 to 2. Mitchell Sharp remained opposed to the scheme and, during 1967, continued to speak publicly about detrimental effects on taxation levels, the economy, and the budget. He predicted that Medicare would cost $1 billion in its first year and would require increased taxation rates equivalent to 12 per cent of personal income tax. The *Globe and Mail* reported that Mr Sharp 'appeared to put the estimate of the cost of medicare in the most dramatic – and frightening – terms possible ... His prime purpose appeared to be to pressure the Cabinet into a review of its determination to press ahead' (18 November 1967: 1). At a Cabinet meeting two days after this announcement, Mitchell Sharp was defeated. A group of pro-Medicare ministers stood behind the prime minister, and the commencement date of 1 July 1968 was confirmed (Taylor 1978: 374).

When the program began, only Saskatchewan and British Columbia were operating schemes that were eligible for cost-sharing. The groups opposing Medicare now concentrated their efforts at the provincial level of government, but, although there was tension, there were no further doctor's strikes, except in Quebec (see below). By January 1971, two and a half years after the commencement date, all provinces had introduced universal medical-insurance plans.

The introduction of Medicare in Quebec deserves special mention because another 'demonstration effect' was created. The government of Saskatchewan had had to concede the right of doctors to set their own fees and to 'opt out' of the insurance plan, billing their patients directly. The federal government's Medical Care Act did not prevent doctors from charging fees to patients but suggested that fees were acceptable only if they did not impede access to necessary medical services, especially for low-income groups (Brown 1983: 46). Outside Quebec, arrangements very similar to those of Saskatchewan were adopted. A politically favourable set of circumstances, however, enabled Quebec to succeed where Saskatchewan had failed.

Medicare in Quebec

At the time of the federal medical-insurance cost-sharing offer, political, social, and economic conditions in Quebec were changing profoundly.[8] There was widespread support for increased government intervention in many aspects of social and economic life, and an activist Liberal government had been in power for five years. It responded to the federal offer by appointing a research committee under the chairmanship of an actuary, Claude Castonguay, to make proposals concerning a medical-insurance system for the province. In 1966, the Liberal government was defeated, but the new government set up another commission of inquiry, again under the chairmanship of Castonguay, to study the entire health-and-welfare system of the province. The commission was asked to give priority to the question of medical insurance and, in 1967, recommended in its first report that a universal, compulsory medical-insurance program be introduced. The scheme was to be financed by an income-related tax (Lee 1979: 7).

Because of financial problems, the government of Quebec wanted to introduce medical insurance in stages, but the conditions attached to the federal offer precluded this approach. Attempts to have the federal government alter the terms of acceptance failed. Finally, in 1969, with an election approaching and both the Liberal opposition and the new Parti Québécois (PQ) pressing for decisive action, the government decided to accept the federal offer. Bill 8 was introduced into the legislature in March. Under the provisions of this legislation, physicians would be able to 'opt out' of the insurance plan, but the patients of these doctors would not be entitled to any reimbursement for the cost of services. The bill was still before the legislature when the government lost office in April 1970.

Bill 8 was revised by the new government and, as a small concession to the medical profession, allowance was made for up to 3 per cent of physicians in any specialty and up to 3 per cent of doctors in any region to opt out of the insurance plan without patients losing the right to reimbursement (Lee 1979: 19–20).

Responses to Bill 8 were varied. The association of general practitioners (FMOQ) approved of the proposals, but the association of specialists (FMSQ) expressed strong disapproval and demanded that the percentage of doctors permitted to opt out be greatly increased. The 'Common Front' of labour, teachers', and farmers' unions strongly opposed the legislation. It was claimed that the bill had been drafted in accordance with the preferences of the medical profession and that it would perpetuate 'intolerable privileges.' Opting-out would lead to two classes of doctors, the unions argued, one class for the rich and another for the poor. They demanded that opting-out be entirely prohibited and that fee-for-service payment be replaced by salary.

Both the FMSQ and the unions threatened strike action if the legislation were not amended. The specialists launched a massive publicity campaign while the general practitioners took the opportunity to negotiate separately with the government. Their main objective was to gain a scale of fees on a uniform basis with specialists for the same services. Under the circumstances, the government's prior intention to selectively negotiate methods of remuneration other than fee-for-service was abandoned (Lee 1979: 17–21).

The position of the FMSQ was not as strong as that of the Saskatchewan doctors had been a decade earlier where the opposition party had supported the profession in its campaign against the government. The threat of strike action was also less effective because general-practitioner services would still be available. Moreover, the FMSQ was strongly opposed by other powerful unions. Nevertheless, the prospect that the province might lose many of its specialists was a strong bargaining lever.

In August 1970, the FMSQ held a mass rally at which 98.5 per cent of specialists determined to 'resort to confrontation' if necessary. This action met with very unfavourable press coverage (*Globe and Mail* 28 August 1970: 1, 3). Despite the low level of support for the FMSQ, the government offered small concessions on the proposed opting-out arrangements. The offer was not accepted. By 5 October 1970, three-quarters of the specialists had left the province (Lee 1979: 21). Further concessions were offered in relation to remuneration, and the government made arrangements for a special sitting of the National Assembly for the following week to effect the necessary amendments in the legislation (Taylor 1978: 407).

The strike was potentially serious because hospital emergency services, normally provided by specialists rather than general practitioners, were disrupted. This crisis, however, was overtaken by another of more serious proportions. The Front de Libération du Québec (FLQ) first kidnapped British diplomat James Cross, and then kidnapped and subsequently murdered deputy premier and minister of Labour Pierre Laporte. Amid fears of insurrection, appeals were made to the specialists to return to work. They refused. An emergency session of the National Assembly was held on 15 October. Under the War Measures Act, the FLQ was outlawed. Medicare was authorized to begin operation on 1 November, whether the FMSQ agreed or not, and the specialists were ordered to return to work. Initially, the association voted to defy the order but, three days later, at the Ottawa headquarters of the CMA, which was guarded by the army, specialists decided reluctantly to go back to work.

Under the amended legislation, opting-out was permitted but patients of non-participating doctors were not entitled to reimbursement from the Insurance Board. Only about ten specialists chose not to join the insurance plan (Lee 1979: 21). Although the government had not been able to negotiate changes in the fee-for-service system of physician remuneration, in these extraordinary circumstances it had succeeded in gaining a very large measure of control over the level of medical fees. The cost of medical services was predictable, and patients were not required to pay a fee at the point of service.

The federal system thus provided an opportunity for the government of Quebec to advance a step farther in terms of achieving social-democratic objectives. Ottawa had set the minimum conditions, and other provinces had not pressed the issue farther. In the late 1970s and early 1980s, opting-out and extra-billing became highly controversial issues, creating serious political difficulties for most governments and giving rise to intense federal-provincial conflict.[9] It was claimed that the principles of Medicare were being eroded, as an increasing number of doctors opted out and charged patients direct fees. Critics were able to point to the Quebec system to support their arguments.

Conclusion

Contrary to 'orthodox' ideas about policy making in federal states, Canadian governments were not weak and conservative in the development of a national health-insurance system. Where activist governments were elected in Saskatchewan and Quebec, these governments vigorously pursued their policies and were willing to undertake the political risks of confrontation with powerful opposing groups, particularly the medical profession. When the Liberal party was committed to reform, as in British Columbia in the 1930s or at the federal level in the 1960s, it too was actively interventionist, although in both cases the opposition of some government members was a constraint on action. The King and St Laurent Liberal governments of the 1940s and 1950s resisted pressures for health and other social-policy reforms, but such resistance was not the result of institutional arrangements. Rather, these governments were conservative in ideology and preferred to follow traditional and cautious economic policies. Nor was federalism the reason that there was little government intervention in health policy in the eastern and central provinces prior to the 1950s. It was simply that no governments committed to social-democratic reform were elected. Some provincial governments were 'bastions of conservatism' but others strongly promoted collectivist policies.

Health-policy development in Canada thus provides little support for the main contentions of traditional federal theories but does lend weight to the 'revisionist' model. At a time when there was little interest in health policy at either the federal level or in other parts of the country, innovations in the western provinces demonstrated that health insurance was administratively and financially feasible, and very popular. The western provinces, the CCF, and other interested groups were able to use provincial experience to press a reluctant federal government into action. Had policy been the sole responsibility of the King and St Laurent governments, the introduction of hospital insurance seems likely to have been delayed for much longer. Canadian experience thus supports Trudeau's argument that federalism may allow regional innovations that can later spread to be made at the regional level under favourable political conditions. It also supports his contention that the division of political and constitutional power does not diminish the sum of government power: national health insurance was introduced through the cumulative efforts of both levels of government. Indeed the division of responsibility enabled Quebec, again under favourable conditions, to take policy a step farther than the rest of the country had taken it in terms of eliminating financial barriers to access to health services.

There is no evidence that the Canadian medical profession was more able to influence policy because power is divided between eleven different governments. Federalism certainly provides multiple access points through which groups can attempt to influence policy but the opportunity to influence does not necessarily provide the capacity to do so. The medical profession was most successful when policies were new and not in operation elsewhere, as in British Columbia in the 1930s and Saskatchewan in the early 1960s. Although no definite causal link can be established, the evidence suggests that the demonstration effect created in the west undermined the profession's position. The Royal Commission on Health Services reported that its findings were influenced by the success of the programs then in operation. After the CMA's failure to prevent the passage of the federal Medical Care Act in 1966, the political struggle continued in the provinces but the profession was unable to prevent the province-by-province spread of the program. And had policy been orchestrated entirely in Ottawa, Quebec doctors would have retained the same billing rights as their counterparts elsewhere.

Thus, contrary to strongly held views in Australia, the development of Canadian health insurance shows that the centralization of power is not necessary to achieve social-policy reforms. The provinces used their constitutional power, and the federal government its financial power and its power to attach conditions to its grants, to facilitate reforms. The five national conditions created enough policy uniformity for insurance cover to be portable between provinces. In this way, ten independent provincial plans were melded by federal participation into a national health-insurance system.

3

Health Services in Australia:
White Settlement to 1950

Health policy in Canada has been concerned primarily with instituting a means of removing financial barriers to access to privately provided health services. Governments[1] have not generally been involved in the direct provision of services or in the administration of health-service institutions.

Australian experience has been quite different. From the early days of white settlement, governments provided health services to varying proportions of the population through institutions that they either operated or subsidized substantially. Whereas in Canada the history of health policy is primarily the history of the development of national health insurance, the focus of early Australian policy was the public provision of services.

In the first half of the century, Commonwealth-government involvement in health was confined to matters of quarantine and, after the establishment of a federal health department in 1921, to the provision of public health services in cooperation with the states. During this time, all states assumed a high level of responsibility for hospital services. Medical care was available in the outpatients departments of public hospitals. Inevitably there were variations in the level of public responsibility in the six states. Some governments were highly interventionist, pursuing policies intended to provide universal and, in some cases, free access to a comprehensive range of health services. The hospitals of Tasmania, for example, were nationalized in 1918, thirty years before nationalization in Britain.

During the world-wide surge of interest in social-policy reform in the 1940s, the federal government became involved in policy making for the provision of personal health services. The proposals put forward were an extension of previous developments in the more radical states. It was envisaged that governments would assume complete responsibility for the provision of all health services, which were to be universally available and free to all citizens. The organization and distribution of a comprehensive range of services was to be planned in detail. Four decades later, only Britain, Sweden, and Quebec in the non-socialist world have attempted such extensive government intervention in the health-care system.

In the development of state policies and in the formulation of plans for a national health service, the Labor party played a crucial role. Except in Tasmania, where non-Labor also extended public responsibility for health care, all major policy innovations were made during periods of Labor government. Like the CCF-NDP in Canada, Labor was successful in placing the issue of universal access to health services on the political agenda. In other respects, however, the impact of Canadian and Australian political parties on policy development was very different. Whereas both the Liberal party and the Progressive Conservative party eventually supported, or acquiesced in, the development of policies formulated by the CCF-NDP, the Australian non-Labor parties have consistently opposed Labor schemes. The non-Labor preference for minimum government intervention in health and the support these parties have given to the medical profession have been among the most important determinants of Australian health policy.

Developments in Britain and in New Zealand also influenced the shape of the Australian health system. In contrast, Canadian developments were more influenced by the different tradition that prevailed in North America. This chapter traces the development of government responsibility for health services in the states and examines the formulation and implementation of policies in the period of joint federal-state activity in the 1940s. The evidence shows a high level of government cooperation both before and after the Commonwealth gained concurrent powers in health.

The Influence of Tradition

Early developments in Australian health policy were very different from those in Canada because ideas in the two countries were based upon different philosophical approaches to health care. Australian developments were influenced by the European tradition in which access to care had come to be considered a right by the end of the nineteenth century. In contrast, Canada followed the American tradition in which the belief that health was a private matter persisted for much longer. These different approaches were noted by Burdett, who observed in 1893 that 'the majority of the population in England consider it not only not a disgrace but the most natural thing in the world, when they fall ill, to demand and receive free treatment without question or delay.' At the same time, he recorded that 'there is relatively little free medical relief anywhere in America ... Americans hold rightly that no person is entitled to occupy a free bed unless or until he can prove beyond dispute that he is unable to pay something for the treatment he receives in the hospital ward' (Burdett 1893: 55–6, quoted in Abel-Smith 1972: 220).

These contrasting ideas are reflected in the different histories of hospital development on the two continents. In many European countries, the provision of hospital services became a public responsibility in the nineteenth century; this increasingly became the case in Britain (Abel-Smith 1972: 220–1). Australia followed the British tradition and developed a network of public and publicly subsidized hospitals. In Canada and in the United States, in contrast, most hospitals were privately owned and managed throughout the nineteenth century.

Public hospitals needed the services of doctors in order to provide medical care for the poor and for low-income earners. Consequently, there emerged in Britain and in Australia a class of hospital-based doctors, some of whom were paid by salary and some of whom gave their services 'gratuitously.' By 1940–1, 60 per cent of the medical staff of Queensland hospitals were paid by salary. The proportions were 37 per cent in Tasmania and between 20 and 25 per cent in the other four Australian states (Brown 1983: 62).

Another important difference between Australia and Canada was that friendly societies or lodges in the European tradition developed in the former but not in the latter. These mutual-benefit organizations provided a means for the prepayment of medical services for low-income earners. In 1913, 46 per cent of the Australian population were eligible to receive medical services from lodge doctors who were engaged by the societies on a contract basis and remunerated by means of capitation payments or, occasionally, by salary.[2] Thus, the private fee-for-service sector of medical practice was relatively small in Australia. The proposals of the 1940s aimed to extend to all citizens the services already available to the poor and to low-income groups, whereas in Canada the policy objective was to provide universal access to privately produced services previously available only to the wealthier members of society. In both health-care systems, the imprint of the past is still apparent. In Canada, there have been few attempts to provide direct services outside Quebec. In Australia, the public provision of services as well as the threat that this presents to the size of the private medical market has been the most contentious issue in health politics for a century.

The Australian Public-Hospital System

The first hospitals in Australia were set up to care for convicts. The premises, equipment, and doctors' salaries were provided by the British government. Free settlers were entitled to treatment, for which no charges were made until 1839, but were reluctant to enter these institutions. Voluntary organizations responded by establishing hospitals for middle-income earners who could not afford private treatment in their own homes (Hospitals and Health Services Commission [HHSC] 1978: 108–10) but from the beginning these organizations were heavily dependent on government subsidization. The Australian public hospital was, therefore, a composite of the types of hospitals that emerged in Britain in the nineteenth century. It combined the characteristics of the tax-financed municipal hospital, which ministered to the poor, with those of the voluntary hospital, which provided for low- and middle-income earners (Brown 1983: 20). In New South Wales and Victoria, hospitals were run by independent boards until the 1920s, despite a level of government subsidy that met more than half of capital and maintenance costs in New South Wales by the 1860s. In the other four states, government provided even larger subsidies and consequently took a larger role in management (Dickey 1980: 41–4; Sax 1984: 25).

In the early nineteenth century Australian hospitals were dirty, ill-equipped, and overcrowded, characteristics that they shared with similar European institutions of the time (Sax 1984: 24). After 1860, in both Britain and Australia there was considerable agitation for reform. Extensive improvements were made, in accordance with 'middle-class notions of respectable civilisation' and ideas about what was 'decently proper for the lower orders' (Dickey 1980: 72).

As hospitals improved and as advances in medical science were made, more and more people came to demand access to treatment. Private hospital owners were not prepared to invest the necessary money in expensive new equipment, and people began to realize that middle- and high-income earners were 'debarred from the most efficient and effective treatment' by the imposition of a means test (Brown 1951: 40–1). Increased demand for admittance created pressure on hospital finances. Governing boards sought to increase voluntary subscriptions in 'an unedifying scramble for money,' but with limited success. Dependence on government funding increased, and hospitals began the practice of admitting patients who could afford to pay at least part of the cost of hospital care (Dickey 1980: 132–6; Thame 1974: 259–60). These changes threatened to erode the size of the private medical market.

The Medical Profession and Australian Public Hospitals

From at least 1890 Australian doctors were concerned with what was termed 'hospital abuse.' Such abuse occurred when those whom physicians suspected were able to pay private medical fees could obtain free care in public hospitals. Almost a century later, the medical profession is still fighting to limit the number of people treated in public wards of public hospitals. In response to the situation in Victoria in 1890, a Melbourne doctor wrote that 'the worst feature of the whole business is the fact that a large section of the community regard [sic] hospitals as institutions put up and maintained for the benefit of anybody who can obtain admission ... There is no realisation of the fact that hospitals are institutions maintained by the benevolence of the public and the profession for paupers ... those who can afford donations, who belong to lodges or are in receipt of fair wages should be rigidly excluded' (*Australian Medical Gazette* [AMG] 15 May 1890: 199).

Although many doctors were not paid for the medical services rendered to hospital patients, there were advantages in hospital work. Appointment to the honorary staff showed that a doctor had risen to a position of some eminence within the profession. Hospital work provided valuable experience and patients who could be used for teaching purposes. Moreover, staff appointments were often stepping-stones to positions as clinical teachers in medical schools. The profession supported the retention of this system but was vehemently opposed to its expansion. A larger public-hospital sector meant either that more services would be provided free or that hospitals would employ more salaried medical practitioners.

Physician opposition to the expansion of the public-hospital system was exacerbated in the early years of the century when the Labor party began to call for the nationalization of hospitals and for free care for all. The profession argued that the employment of salaried staff would lower standards of care and would exclude from hospital work 'experienced and matured practitioners whose services the governments could not possibly afford to command' (*Medical Journal of Australia* [MJA] 22 April 1916: 343–4; 12 May 1917: 409).

The solution that finally emerged and that gained acceptance in the 1920s and 1930s was the development of community hospitals along American lines. Intermediate and private wards were added to public hospitals and doctors were able to charge fees to non-public patients. However, if this system were to operate to the satisfaction of the profession, access to public wards had to be controlled. Despite the enduring opposition of the profession, especially in New South Wales and Victoria, considerable progress was made in providing hospital services for increasing numbers of people. This trend culminated in a universal 'free' hospital system, introduced in 1946, that completely altered the original 'charitable' basis of the provision of hospital services. Prior to the introduction of this system, however, Australian state governments developed a variety of policy responses to the growing demand for hospital care.

Public Hospitals in the States

A compromise acceptable to the medical profession and to government in relation to hospital care appears to have been worked out in South Australia and Western Australia in the early years of the century. In both states, there were government hospitals and government-subsidized hospitals. South Australia began to admit fee-paying patients before the turn of the century, a practice introduced in Western Australia in the 1920s. Hospitals were staffed by a mixture of honorary, full-time, and part-time medical practitioners. No medical fees were charged to patients in government hospitals but, in subsidized hospitals, patients who could afford to pay medical fees were permitted to do so. In both states, by 1941–2, well over 90 per cent of hospital-maintenance costs came from combined government subsidy and patient payments (MJA 31 August 1929: 298–9; Thame 1974: 260–5; Joint Committee on Social Security [JCSS] 1944: 9).

The charitable element in the provision of hospital services was stronger, and survived longer in Victoria than in any other state. In 1931, donations still provided almost one-third of hospital revenues but had fallen to 16 per cent by 1941–2 (Dampney 1951 appendix 1: 2; JCSS 1944: 9). Large metropolitan hospitals were less reliant on government funds than average figures indicate and these institutions retained considerable independence. Although it was agreed that more hospitals for paying patients were needed, there was wide support for the idea that this expansion should be achieved with minimum government intervention.

In other states, as in England, an alternative set of proposals emerged in the early years of the century. It was argued, mainly by representatives of the labour movement, that tax-financed hospitals, accessible to all without charge or means test, should be established. The Victorian Labor party did not adopt these ideas as readily as its counterparts in other states, and neither Labor nor non-Labor governments attempted to take full control of Victorian public hospitals (Inglis 1958: 177–80).

Nevertheless, after several abortive attempts, a Victorian non-Labor government sufficiently overcame the forces of voluntarism to pass the Hospitals and Charities Act in 1922. A charities board to act as a mediator between hospitals and the government was established with wide powers to intervene in the management, closure, amalgamation, and establishment of hospitals and to allocate subsidies to different institutions (MJA 31 August 1929: 295–7; Inglis 1958: 183–7). By the early 1940s, Victorian hospitals were required to abide by a growing number of conditions set down by the board in order to be eligible for grants. Thus, although the degree of government control that had developed in other states was 'unknown in Victoria,' the trend was towards increased intervention in the organization and provision of hospital services.

The first attempt to introduce the Labor alternative of public provision of a comprehensive range of health services was made by the McGowan government, elected in New South Wales in 1910. The minister responsible for health services was the Hon. Fred Flowers (1864–1928), first in his capacity as acting chief secretary and later as minister for the newly established Department of Public Health. Health services had been discussed at Labor party conferences for some years. As early as 1898, the Political Labor League had included in its platform a proposal to divide 'the country into medical districts in charge of competent medical officers whose services shall be absolutely free' (Political Labor League 1898, The Platform). By 1908, the League had formulated proposals for the provision of a comprehensive range of hospital and medical services, which included universal access to free hospital care (HHSC 1978: 111; Dickey 1976: 60). In 1911, Flowers argued that 'hospitals are a necessity of civilisation and the Government should see to their upkeep and control. Hospitals should be as free as the Art Gallery or the Public Library ... and there should be no taint of pauperism' (quoted in Dickey 1976: 62–3).

The local branch of the British Medical Association in Australia (BMA)[3] completely opposed these ideas and called for increased philanthropic support to enable hospitals to dispense with government aid (AMG 20 November 1911: 679–80). The profession was supported by the non-Labor party, by hospital boards, and by the Shires Association, which itself wanted to take control of country hospitals. In the event, no concrete plans for the nationalization of hospitals were put forward during Labor's term of office. The government had only a narrow majority in the Legislative Assembly and did not control the Legislative Council. After protracted negotiations with doctors, pharmacists, and some friendly societies, the government was forced to abandon its proposals to establish free general dispensaries.

Nevertheless, progress was made in reforming existing institutions and in establishing new services. Subsidies were increased and grants to extend facilities were made. Government asylums were expanded and improved so that, in effect, they became hospitals rather than asylums. The government hospital at Little Bay was upgraded and expanded to become the largest hospital in the state and was opened to all citizens. Convalescent homes were built, tuberculosis clinics were established, and subsidies for sanatoria were made available. A maternity scheme was launched in 1912, homes for mothers and babies were provided, and the visiting-nurse service was extended. A school medical service was set up in 1912 and extended to country areas in 1913. In order to augment services in country areas, the work of the Bush Nursing Association was supported in a variety of ways. Responsibility for all health services, which had previously been divided among different departments, was given to the new Department of Public Health, established in 1914 (Dickey 1976: 68–70). These reforms were part of a comprehensive plan for the 'Nationalisation of Public Health' adopted at the Political Labor Conference in 1912 and were very similar to the proposals for a national health service that the federal Labor governments of the 1940s attempted to implement. The New South Wales system was to be financed from consolidated revenue, and doctors were to be paid by salary (AMG 10 February 1912: 134–5).

After Flowers's failure to gain control of the public-hospital system, developments in New South Wales paralleled those in Victoria. A hospitals commission was established in 1929, with wider powers than its Victorian counterpart (Inglis 1958: 189). Hospital facilities were improved, and fee-setting was regularized. As in Victoria, a hospital-building program began in the mid-1930s, and intermediate and private wings were added to the public hospitals (Thame 1974: 285).

Tasmania was the first state to eliminate the charitable basis of the provision of hospital services. After a protracted and bitter struggle between both Labor and non-Labor governments and the medical profession, the government took control of hospital boards in 1918. During the dispute, in which two royal commissions were held, the honorary staff at the major hospitals tendered their resignations. The government's response was to appoint salaried medical officers, some of whom were BMA members, without delay. Under the new arrangements introduced in 1918, medical need alone became the criterion for determining eligibility for hospital care, and after this time no person was denied admission by reason of inability to pay. Neither subscribers (of whom there were few) nor doctors were represented on hospital boards, where government nominees formed a majority. The provision of private accommodation in public hospitals was prohibited.[4]

Although acrimonious negotiations continued over the question of medical practice in hospitals, successive Tasmanian governments vigorously pursued a policy that provided universal access to single-standard hospital care according to people's ability to pay.[5] In achieving these objectives, governments were greatly aided by the fact that the BMA could not control all of its members. Had the government of 1917 been unable to attract salaried hospital doctors, it would almost certainly have been forced to accede to some of the BMA's demands.

The nationalization of hospitals and the abolition of the honorary system was also undertaken in Queensland, and was achieved during a long period of Labor rule. The party held power from 1915 until 1957, with an interruption of only three years during the depression. At the Labor-in-Politics Convention in 1905, the nationalization of hospitals was adopted as part of the platform. The development of hospital policy involved a long political struggle between Labor and non-Labor: Labor wanted to levy a hospital maintenance tax on landowners whereas non-Labor wanted a tax on income and wages.

Legislation designed to relieve a financial crisis facing the Brisbane Hospital was introduced in 1905 but was rejected by the Legislative Council (Leggett 1976: 9–29).[6] By 1915 it was realized that voluntary donations could not be relied upon to meet even part of hospital costs. Further legislation was introduced in 1916–17, again designed to shift some of the responsibility onto local government, but was again rejected by the landowner-dominated Upper House (Bell 1976: 287–8). In the meantime, the financial situation of the Brisbane hospital became critical. The board resigned, and the former secretary was engaged to manage the hospital on behalf of the Home Secretary's Department (*MJA* April 1917: 307; *Brisbane Courier* 3 April 1917: 6).

After the abolition of the Legislative Council in 1922, the government began preparation for hospital reform so that 'the workers of Queensland would no longer have to depend on charity for their health services' (Bell

1976: 288). A system of 'districting' was introduced, and area boards were set up. Hospital deficits were met by state and local government on a 60–40 basis. The reforms were based upon the system in operation in New Zealand and were influenced by the recommendations of one of the Tasmanian royal commissions (Leggett 1976: xviii–xix, 31–2).

For the rest of the 1920s, there was strong opposition to the land tax. In some cases, conflict erupted between the area boards and honorary medical officers who were pressing for the development of non-public hospital wards. In 1930, the non-Labor government appointed a royal commission to inquire into the hospital system. Recommendations were made for a tax on wages, salaries, and incomes, but no action was taken because of the political difficulty of introducing another tax during the depression. Under continued pressure from the BMA, a small number of intermediate beds were introduced into public hospitals in the 1930s but no private beds were permitted (Leggett 1976: 32–56).

Labor returned to office in 1932 and set up the Department of Health and Home Affairs. Health, hospitals, and local government were combined in one portfolio, under E.M. Hanlon, who later became treasurer, and then premier. Another Hospitals Act was passed in 1936, ostensibly to give boards greater control over hospitals, but the real effect was to give the government greater control over boards (Bell 1976: 291). An inspector of hospitals was appointed, and boards were empowered to provide services in a wide range of areas, including dentistry, maternal and child welfare, mental illness, and optometry, and to provide ambulance and transport services. The act provided that the chairman of each board would be a government appointee and that ministerial approval was needed for the appointment of hospital superintendents. With the intention of creating a full-time salaried medical service, boards were given the power to employ doctors instead of making honorary appointments. Under this provision, the honorary staff of Brisbane Hospital were replaced in 1938. The act also prohibited the establishment of new voluntary hospitals (Leggett 1976: 57–89).

The final stage in the long process of nationalization took place in 1944 in anticipation of the free national hospital scheme that was about to be introduced. The state government took full responsibility for all hospital finances and, from 1 July 1945, all inpatient and outpatient services were made available to all citizens without charge.

Thus where Flowers had failed to take control of the hospital system in New South Wales, the governments of Queensland and Tasmania had succeeded. The opposition of the medical profession was the most

important obstacle in each state. In the same way that the profession opposed government control of the hospital system, it opposed the development of other government health services because these, too, were seen
as a threat to the size of the private medical market.

State Health Services and the Medical Profession

After 1850, there had been an expansion of state-government activity from
the original public-health services, such as sanitation and food inspection, into areas of preventive and social medicine (Dampney 1951: 6, 1).
The Commonwealth entered the public-health area after the establishment of the Department of Health in 1921. In cooperation with the states,
public-health services were developed and expanded, although expenditure restraint during the depression placed limits on the extent to which
proposals were implemented. The medical profession accepted the provision of public-health services but was opposed to any service that provided care for the individual during 'sickness, injury or childbirth' (MJA
27 February 1915: 195). With varying degrees of intensity in different
states, doctors resisted the expansion of services that might become a substitute for private medical care.

Infant-welfare services were first established in Sydney in the early
years of the century and, in another example of the 'demonstration effect,' quickly spread to other states. These services were extended by the
New South Wales Labor government after 1912. The medical profession
was not at first opposed to these developments but, by 1916, doctors 'were
seeking assurances that only the indigent would be permitted to attend,
that the service would be restricted to infants under one year of age, that
no treatment would be given and that no nurse would visit the home of
a mother not under the care of a doctor' (Sax 1984: 18). Infant-welfare
centres provided services free of charge and were gradually taken advantage of by mothers of all income groups. However, the medical profession succeeded in restricting the range of services that were available.

Another innovation in New South Wales was the establishment of a
night clinic at the Royal Prince Alfred Hospital for the treatment of vene-
real disease. The clinic attracted hundreds of patients in its first few days
of operation but was opposed by the profession: doctors feared that people who could afford to pay private fees might receive free treatment. As
it had with the infant-welfare services, the profession demanded that only
the poor be allowed to attend (MJA 24 April 1915: 382–4).

The development of school health services was also retarded by medical opposition. Introduced in Tasmania and Western Australia in 1907, these schemes expanded slowly, partly because some governments were reluctant to provide sufficient funds and partly because the profession refused to countenance the development of comprehensive services (Thame 1974: 215–39). The inspection of children for defects was accepted reluctantly but treatment of the many problems that such inspections uncovered was opposed vehemently. When the New South Wales government found itself unable to expand the service in 1916 because doctors were unwilling to join, it threatened to send to China for physicians. The *MJA* confidently predicted that the government would not be able to recruit the necessary staff and said that the minister would have to accept the profession's conditions (2 September 1916: 186). There were only thirty-nine full-time school doctors in Australia in 1943, when it was estimated that four times the number were needed to provide an annual examination for all schoolchildren (Thame 1974: 238).

Other services affected similarly were industrial hygiene, maternal welfare, and the Bush Nursing Service. The restricted development of health services not only was a result of active opposition but also followed from the failure of doctors to act as a force for change and reform. As Thame has argued 'because it was against the interests of the profession to undermine private practice, those members of the community best equipped to provide governments with convincing arguments for the mass treatment and prevention of disease were precisely those who did not do so, except for a few dedicated public health officers who swam against the tide of medical opinion' (1974: 238–9). If there were doctors who were opposed to the position taken by the leaders of the BMA, their opinions were rarely published in the pages of the *MJA*. An exception was Dr A.E. Brown of Victoria, who was concerned about public perceptions of 'a medical profession jealously watchful of its own interests.' Summarizing the stance the profession had taken towards the non-private health sector, he wrote:

we have allowed every single reform measure to come into being without any aid from us, nor any interest, except such an attitude as the 'armed neutrality' involved in the procedure of 'guarding our interests' ... there is no justification of our attitudes towards such movements as the Bush Nursing and Baby Health Centre Schemes. Granting that some medical men did of their own volition actively interest themselves in the inception of these movements, we as a profession played a very inglorious part in it. And now that they are established we regard them at best with approval, tempered by fear lest they encroach on our medical preserves. At worst, our members show a frank hostility toward them ... (*MJA* 26 February 1927: 298)

Considered in the context of the time, the Australian states had assumed a high level of responsibility for the provision of health services, despite the enduring opposition of the medical profession. The evidence presented here is not consistent with Thame's thesis that 'responsibility for health care remained primarily with the individual during the first half of the twentieth century' (1974: 340). Thame argues that hospitals were thought to be an essential service that had to be provided in all states, 'no matter what else was neglected,' and that state governments were 'forced' to expand services. This argument is itself a recognition that the notion of collective responsibility had come to hold considerable sway. In contrast, such notions were weak in Canada. During the same period, the public provision of hospital services was not considered to be essential and, unlike the case in Australia, government intervention was limited. The Australian situation is better explained by the interaction of two sets of competing forces: the Labor party and the notion of collective responsibility, on the one hand, and the non-Labor parties, the medical profession, and the concept of individual responsibility, on the other.

By 1941–2, Australian public hospitals were providing 60 per cent of all inpatient services in Victoria and South Australia, 67 per cent in New South Wales, 70 per cent in Western Australia, and 80 and 84 per cent in Queensland and Tasmania, respectively. A total of 571 government and subsidized hospitals supplied 73 per cent of Australian hospital beds (JCSS 1943: 54). Hospitals also provided medical services for 18 per cent of the population in public outpatient departments.[7] Finally, the states of Tasmania, Western Australia, and New South Wales had developed a policy of employing salaried doctors in some rural areas to overcome the undersupply of private practitioners.

The National Health Scheme proposals of the Curtin and Chifley governments were not, then, a radical departure from tradition but were rather an expansion and continuation of state policies, particularly those of Labor governments. In fact, there was little advance on the proposals developed in New South Wales by 1912. The ideas of the 1940s were also influenced by a worldwide resurgence of interest in social-policy reform. The leaders of the medical profession, however, had not modified their long-standing opposition to government health services, and the stage was set for a long struggle in which the Commonwealth achieved only some of its objectives despite the cooperative attitude of the states.

Health-Policy Making in the 1940s[8]

The high level of federal-state cooperation in health-policy formulation during the 1940s is perhaps best explained by the predominance of Labor governments in most jurisdictions. Throughout the period, New South Wales, Queensland, and Tasmania were governed by Labor. Victoria had a period of Labor government between 1945 and 1947, and Labor was in power in Western Australia until 1947. Non-Labor governed in South Australia throughout the period, but its premier, Thomas Playford, showed no opposition to the principles of the proposals in discussions at the premiers' conferences of the period. Under these circumstances, policies were implemented through federal-state cooperation and the use of conditional grants to the states.

The Labor party came to power in October 1941 and remained in government until the end of 1949. John Curtin was prime minister until his death in 1945, when he was succeeded by J.B. Chifley. In keeping with tradition, Labor quickly set about the task of trying to gain increased Commonwealth powers.[9] It was proposed that a referendum be held, at which the people should be asked to transfer a total of fourteen powers from the states to the Commonwealth. The states objected to the extent of the proposed transfer, and a constitutional convention was held in 1942, at which a compromise was reached: the federal government would give up its plans for a referendum during the war if the states would agree to transfer the fourteen powers for a period until five years after the end of hostilities. In the event, only New South Wales and Queensland were prepared to transfer the powers in full. Victoria would do so if all other states did, while South Australia and Western Australia passed legislation transferring the powers, but with substantial amendments. Tasmanian legislation was rejected by the Legislative Council.

The Commonwealth then determined to put the fourteen matters to a referendum. During the Commonwealth parliamentary debates on the Referendum Bill, the power of 'national health in cooperation with the states or any one of them' was a non-controversial issue, and no arguments in support of states' rights were put forward. Objections centred upon the perceived socialist potential of the other powers. The referendum of August 1944 failed in all states except South Australia and Western Australia (Hunter 1968: 136–43).

After this setback, the government decided to modify its centralization objectives. In the meantime, the High Court decision in the first *Pharmaceutical Benefits* case in November 1945 cast doubt upon the constitutional validity of other federal social policies, including maternity benefits, widow's pensions, and unemployment and sickness benefits, which all relied on the appropriation power of Section 81. It was decided that the appropriation of money 'for the purposes of the Commonwealth' was invalid if the Commonwealth otherwise lacked the constitutional power to legislate in the area.

The next federal attempt to gain extended powers in 1946 was altogether more limited and, instead of the proposals being 'packaged,' as in 1944, the items were listed separately. This move proved to be politically astute because, in the event, the proposals concerning the marketing of primary products and the power to control industrial employment failed to gain a majority in the necessary fourth state (although a national majority was achieved). The proposal to expand federal-government power for the provision of social services was approved in all states. A new section (51: 23A) was added to the constitution; it empowers the Commonwealth to legislate with respect to 'the provision of maternity allowances, widows' pensions, child endowment, unemployment, pharmaceutical, sickness and hospital benefits, medical and dental services (but not so as to authorise any form of civil conscription), benefits to students and family allowances.' This amendment gave the federal government very wide concurrent powers in relation to health. The term 'benefits' has a broad meaning and allows, as well as cash benefits, benefits in kind and the direct provision of services. It enables the Commonwealth to legislate for the detailed administration of any scheme designed to provide benefits or services and to determine the method of financing (Sackville 1978: 55–6). Moreover, the Commonwealth can establish its own institutions, such as hospitals and pharmacies, if it wishes (Sax 1984: 121).

The clause, 'but not so as to authorise any form of civil conscription,' was a legislative amendment proposed by the leader of the opposition, R.G. Menzies, at the instigation of Sir Henry Newland, president of the Federal Council of the BMA (Scott-Young 1962: 23). Menzies argued that the amendment would be a safeguard against the nationalization of the two professions. The government's acceptance of this amendment is interesting. It had previously rejected two other proposed amendments, one designed to separate health from the other social-service powers and the other to keep health out of the referendum proposals altogether. In this case, the amendment had been circulated for some time and, after consideration, Attorney General Evatt announced that 'if industrial workers are entitled to be protected against conscription, members of the medical and dental professions are entitled to similar protection. I therefore have pleasure in accepting this amendment' (quoted in Hunter 1968: 150).

Hunter finds this decision 'surprising and difficult to explain' in the light of subsequent events. She suggests that the concession may have been considered necessary to ensure the passage of the referendum or to stem 'the rising tide of opposition to Labor's other socialistic policies' (1968: 150–1). Both of these considerations were undoubtedly important, but Evatt's own later explanation that the government did not envisage the use of compulsion is equally important. It is highly unlikely that any government would willingly incur the political costs of attempting to conscript a powerful group such as the medical profession, and it is even more unlikely that a successful medical service could be administered in this way. Thus, the clause has far less practical importance than has often been suggested.

The success of the 1946 constitutional amendment radically altered the federal balance of power in relation to health. It gave the Commonwealth formal power to intervene in almost any aspect of policy. This capacity was enhanced by the centralization of financial power in 1942. However, the impact of the constitutional amendment on health policy in the 1940s was negligible. First, the policies which were implemented successfully came into operation before the passage of the referendum. Second, formal power did not help the government to gain physician support for a national medical service or a pharmaceutical-benefits scheme. Third, the federal government had taken a leadership role in policy development from the beginning of its term of office. Policy makers were aware that even if the Commonwealth failed to gain additional powers, programs could be implemented in cooperation with the states. The broad outlines of most policies put forward after 1946 had already been developed during the war.

Proposals for a National Health Service

Two main bodies were involved in policy making at the federal level in the 1940s. The first was the National Health and Medical Research Council (NHMRC), a federal-state creation on which the BMA, the College of Physicians, the College of Surgeons, the medical schools of Australian universities, and federal and state governments were represented. One of its functions was to provide advice to both levels of government 'on all matters of public health legislation and administration, on matters concerning the health of the public and on medical research.' A considerable program of federal-state activity in public health areas had been developed through the council prior to the war (CPD HR 2 October 1945: 6228).

The second policy-making body was the Joint Committee on Social Security (JCSS). This parliamentary committee was set up by the Menzies government in July 1941 'and was seen as a response to Labor efforts to promote social policy reform' (Hunter 1968: 81). The committee remained in existence until 1946, although there were membership changes. It published nine reports on different aspects of social policy, four of which dealt with health matters.

The Federal Council of the BMA had no definite health policy at this time. Traditionally opposed to health insurance, salaried service, and contract practice, the council struggled to formulate a policy that would extend access to services but at the same time preserve a large sector of private practice. To add to its problems, a subcommittee of the Victorian branch of the BMA formulated a proposal for a salaried service in 1941. There was also strong support in Queensland for this mode of practice. Dr F.L. Davies summarized the policy dilemma at the time when he said that the Federal Council did not know what the profession wanted or what it would be offered (MJA 1 November 1941: 515). The council itself, however, was totally opposed to government-sponsored health services. When the government attempted to implement schemes based on the proposals of the NHMRC, the JCSS, and the health ministers' conferences, it fought hard and successfully to defend private practice.

The NHMRC and a Salaried Medical Service

In May 1941, Sir Frederick Stewart, Minister for Health and long-time campaigner for social insurance (Watts 1983: 113–20), asked the NHMRC to develop recommendations for a possible health scheme. A subcommittee presented a report later in the year, titled *Outline of a Possible Scheme for a Salaried Medical Service*. Although the council stated that its proposals were a framework for discussion rather than a final and complete scheme, a very detailed regionalized system had been worked out. Assessments had been made of facility and staff requirements for every locality in the country. Costs had been estimated, and the details of pay and conditions of service were set out. No recommendation was made about how the scheme should be financed, but the council thought 'some form of direct or indirect taxation' was inevitable. It was recognized that implementation would require 'some modification of the Commonwealth of Australia Constitution Act of 1901' but the council saw 'no insuperable difficulty in complete control by the Commonwealth, even including the transfer of State Health Departments.'[10]

While this opinion was undoubtedly an overly optimistic assessment of the politics of federalism, it does attest to the very low level of state opposition to federal intervention in the health field that prevailed at the time. The reactions of some state politicians to the first policy announcements of the new Labor minister for Health and Social Services, E.J. Holloway, in 1941 confirm that the NHMRC was not out of touch with opinion in at least three states. Tasmanian premier R. Cosgrove told the press that 'the Government believes that it would be better for the Commonwealth to take charge of health matters, provided it took complete charge and instituted a system of free medical services in country districts similar to those operating in Tasmania.' N.S.W. Health minister C.A. Kelly was of the opinion that the health of the community should be a national concern and should be taken over by the federal government. Western Australian Health minister A.H. Panton 'wholeheartedly agreed' that medical services should be nationalized and thought that such should be done on a Commonwealth basis.¹¹ No objections were expressed to the idea of an expanded Commonwealth policy role at the health ministers' and premiers' conferences of the 1940s. Moreover, only Victoria, in the period of non-Labor government, opposed the principle of free health services.

The Proposals of the Joint Committee on Social Security

In 1942, Treasurer Chifley requested the JCSS to report on a system of health services, with particular reference to measures that might be introduced during the war. The committee advised that, in its 'considered opinion,' it would be impossible to introduce a comprehensive scheme during the war. However, it suggested that planning could proceed. It then sought the opinions of a wide range of groups, including state governments and the medical profession. Proposals and plans considered were the NHMRC 'Outline,' the New Zealand health and social security system, and the Beveridge Report. The chairman of the New Zealand Social Security Commission and the secretary of the New Zealand Department of Health were consulted. The concept of health insurance was rejected. The committee argued that 'national Health Insurance has never been part of the health and medical services of this country' (JCSS 1943: 6). The advantages and disadvantages of salary, fee-for-service, and the capitation method of physician remuneration, all of which were operating simultaneously in New Zealand, were examined. It was found that there was opposition and support for all of these systems within the medical profession. However, there was far less opposition to a salaried service if control were vested in the profession through an independent statutory body. The committee recommended as follows:

- a general medical service providing services for the whole community, to be financed from a central fund raised by an income-related tax;
- for remote areas, a full-time, voluntary salaried medical service with improved hospital and transport services;
- for all other areas, a part-time salaried service, where physicians otherwise engaged in private practice would work for a nominated number of half-days per week in specially provided clinics equipped with modern facilities. The control of each clinic would be vested in its medical personnel.

On the question of administrative authority, the committee noted that the scheme could be run by the Commonwealth if the federal government gained the necessary constitutional power, or the Commonwealth might lay down the broad principles of a scheme and provide support to the states by means of Section 96 grants (JCSS 1943).

The *Seventh Interim Report* of the JCSS, presented in February 1944, addressed the question of a Commonwealth hospital-benefits scheme. Three sets of arrangements were considered, but the committee recommended that the Commonwealth pay the states a flat-rate subsidy per daily occupied bed, based upon the amount received from patients' fees. Under this scheme, Victoria, Queensland, and South Australia would accrue a substantial surplus, which was to be paid into a trust fund earmarked for extension and improvement of hospital facilities, a recognition that such an expansion would have to be delayed until wartime shortages had been overcome.[12] By means of the subsidy, the states would be able to offer public-ward accommodation at no charge and would be able to reduce charges to patients in intermediate and private wards of public hospitals by the amount of the subsidy. As with other committee proposals, the scheme was to be financed by an income-related tax paid into a special fund.

The NHMRC proposal of 1941 attracted intense opposition from the BMA. The JCSS was more cautious and took care to consider the profession's evidence. Its proposals represented an attempt to reach a compromise that would attract as much support as possible. It recommended strongly against the early adoption of a comprehensive scheme, which, it argued, would be 'vigourously opposed,' and reminded the government that former Health minister E.J. Holloway had given the BMA an undertaking that no major changes would be introduced during the war or for one year thereafter (JCSS 1943: 19–20).

In 1943, the government announced that it would proceed with its health plans in accordance with the recommendations of the JCSS. Besides the profession's opposition, shortages of health workers and materials imposed restraints. As Minister for Post-War Reconstruction, Chifley realized that many plans would have to wait until after the war. It was decided, however, that the cash-benefits part of social programs could proceed. Chifley believed that if a start were not made in this area during the war 'all sorts of excuses w[ould] be found when the War ends for not passing them' (quoted in Crisp n.d.: 190-1).

Accordingly, a list of priorities[13] was developed among the various health proposals. The stages in the 'evolution of a Commonwealth Medical service' were to be:

1 Pharmaceutical Benefits
2 Hospital Benefits
3 Payment of honoraries in public hospitals with gradual development of salaried specialists
4 Full Diagnostic Laboratories and X-Ray Units in country areas
5 Salaried service in one-man towns[14]
6 Experimental salaried group-practice centres in a number of industrial towns, e.g. Lithgow, Kalgoolie, Port Pirie and Broken Hill[15]
7 Metropolitan areas – establishment of health centres in selected areas
8 Development of salaried medical services in larger country towns
9 Increase of health centres in metropolitan areas and increased use of salaried staff attached to hospitals for all medical work in district, until all necessary medical services are on a salaried basis
10 At a stage to be decided, all medical services to be free

It was estimated that this program could be achieved in stages over a period of seven years after 1945, even with the existing building restrictions and staff training needs.[16] First priority was given to the supply of free medicines, a scheme that did not involve the states but is important in a study of federalism because of the use the medical profession was able to make of the constitution.

The Pharmaceutical-Benefits Scheme

Quite where the original idea to provide free medicines originated remains obscure but policy makers were influenced by both the New Zealand and British schemes then in operation. It was a decision that the government came to regret when the intensity of the opposition of the medical profession became apparent. In 1947, Health minister N.E. McKenna told Cabinet that 'it is certain that if the Commonwealth Government were now embarking upon the field of National Health for the first time, that pharmaceutical benefits would not be introduced as the first, or even one of the first, measures ... [I]t would be allowed to develop gradually.'[17]

Officially, the profession objected to the formulary, which it claimed was not comprehensive enough. It opposed the use of government prescription forms; the inclusion of penalty clauses in the 1944 act, which were intended to control abuse; and the proposed administration by a government department. Concern was also expressed that the scheme might provide an opportunity to introduce a salaried medical service in rural areas 'by the back door.' The real objection appears to have been to the introduction of a free, universal, publicly administered scheme. First, the BMA, while arguing that the proposed formulary was not comprehensive enough, was willing to accept a far more limited list of medicines.[18] Further, in a confidential letter to the director general of Health in November 1948, the president of Federal Council suggested that agreement might be reached if patients were required to pay part of the cost of medicines.[19] Thus if patients had been required to pay and the scheme had been limited, the BMA's objections might have been overcome.

Extensive negotiations were held between 1944 and 1948 but no agreement was reached. The government made some concessions but refused to compromise on the question of the formulary or on the use of government forms. The formulary was a compromise between the limited British list of medicines and the completely unlimited New Zealand list. It had been found that in New Zealand, neither costs nor abuse could be controlled.[20] By June 1948, the profession refused to negotiate further unless the government first agreed to the elimination of government forms, to the removal of all penal clauses, and to the limitation of the formulary.[21] The deadlock was thus complete. In retrospect, it seems highly unlikely that agreement was ever a possibility.

In this part of its health policy, the government left itself open to challenges on constitutional grounds, and the medical profession made full use of this avenue of opposition. The Pharmaceutical Benefits Act 1944 was challenged and declared invalid by the High Court in 1945. This decision was used by the government as a justification for wider Commonwealth powers in social-policy areas. The threat to the validity of existing benefits was, in Sawer's opinion, one reason that the referendum was successful (1963: 219).

After the passage of the referendum, the government passed a second pharmaceutical benefits act in 1947. The BMA advised members not to co-operate and to return the formulary and the prescription forms, which the government had supplied, unopened. Only about 150–200 practitioners disregarded this advice. For eighteen months, doctors refused to abide by the provisions of valid legislation. As the MJA described the situation in 1949: 'the Commonwealth took a referendum from the people on the whole question of social services and was granted constitutional powers to legislate in such matters. But this was of little avail because, although the Pharmaceutical Benefits Act was passed and received Royal Assent, the medical profession opposed it on ethical grounds and on the question of freedom and refused to cooperate. The Pharmaceutical Benefits Act is now dead as a dodo' (MJA 5 February 1949: 160).

It was the government's attempt to force the profession to abide by the legislation that gave rise to the second challenge. The 1947 act was amended to make it an offence for a medicine included in the formulary to be written on a non-government prescription form. The amendment was challenged and declared unconstitutional in October 1949. The act itself remained valid.

Had the profession's challenge been unsuccessful, the government would have been forced to resort to the mass prosecution of doctors to gain compliance with the act. But 1949 was an election year and opinion had begun to turn against the government. The opposition, the medical profession, and other groups such as the banks were campaigning against Labor policies on grounds that they would lead to a restriction of liberty and would promote the 'Red Menace' and 'crypto-Fascism' (Bolton 1974: 493–503). One journalist commented that public opinion was not so much 'behind the doctors' as 'indifferent.'[22] Under these circumstances, the enforcement of legal sanctions would have been a politically risky venture. On only one occasion in both Canada and Australia has a government chosen to use legal coercion to gain the 'cooperation' of the medical profession. The Quebec government was able to order specialists to return to work, but, as we saw in chapter 2, the prevailing political conditions were extraordinarily favourable. It is unlikely that the Australian government could have forced the profession to participate in its free-medicine scheme, even in the absence of the constitutional clause prohibiting the civil conscription of doctors and dentists. As Dampney argued in 1951, 'by a strategy of non-cooperation and delay, the profession was able to drive the government beyond its constitutional limits and then appeal to the High Court to proclaim the unvalidity of the measures' (Dampney 1951: 7, 24).

The Hospital-Benefits Scheme

The second program on the government's list of health priorities was a hospital-benefits scheme. Before September 1946, the Commonwealth had no constitutional power in relation to hospitals. However, a system of free hospital care was introduced in cooperation with the states. Importantly, the Commonwealth did not need to negotiate with the Federal Council of the BMA.

After preliminary talks between federal and state officials, it was decided that regular Commonwealth–State health ministers' conferences should be held, and the first of these took place in June 1943. The Seventh Interim Report of the JCSS was presented in February 1944. In the following July the health ministers met again, this time with federal treasurer Ben Chifley present. Proposals for a hospital-benefits scheme, drafted by the Commonwealth on the basis of the JCSS report, were put before the conference. In the meantime at the January 1944 Premiers' Conference it was agreed unanimously that the financing of the decisions of the ministers for Health should be a joint Commonwealth–State responsibility.[23]

Not all state health ministers agreed with all aspects of the hospital-benefits proposals. Queensland, Tasmania, and Western Australia supported the provision of free public-ward care, and the South Australian minister saw no problem in presenting the plan to his government. New South Wales thought there would be a heavy demand for free care and wanted to retain a means test to direct the wealthy to intermediate and private wards. Mr Chifley thought that those who could afford it would continue to choose private accommodation and observed that it was in the interests of doctors that there be as many private patients as possible. After discussion, the decision to provide free treatment in public wards was taken. Only the Victorian minister did not endorse the agreement. Once certain standards had been established, the administration of the scheme was to be left to the states.[24]

The scheme was approved by federal Cabinet the following week, after which the prime minister wrote to the premiers, making a formal proposal. The matter was discussed at the Premiers' Conference held in August 1944, where again some objections were raised by some states, chiefly New South Wales and Victoria. The New South Wales government had very little to gain financially because the difference between the federal subsidy and the amount being collected in fees was only threepence per patient per day.[25] Victoria remained opposed to the principle of the scheme. Both states reported that hospital associations and hospital boards opposed the proposals, and the question of whether the medical profession would continue to provide honorary services became an issue. Despite objections, the terms of the prime minister's formal offer were accepted.[26]

After the Premiers' Conference, work on administrative details proceeded at officer level. The main problem concerned the payment of honorary doctors. Victoria refused to furnish statistics until the Commonwealth undertook to reimburse the states for paying doctors, should honoraries withdraw their services. Western Australia voiced similar concerns.[27] The Commonwealth agreed to the reimbursement proposal, and a hospital benefits act was passed in October 1945. The means test was abolished in all hospitals in 1946, and hospital care was available free to all who chose public-ward accommodation. The Commonwealth paid the states a subsidy of six shillings per occupied bed day for all approved hospitals, both public and private. The fees charged to private patients were reduced by the amount of the federal subsidy.[28] In the event, only Tasmanian honoraries chose to accept payment for their services. The decentralized administration of the scheme proved to be 'quite satisfactory.'[29]

There were several reasons that the hospital-benefits scheme was introduced without serious political difficulty. In the first place, Labor was in power in five of the six states in 1945–6. Second, the scheme had implications only for hospital-based doctors. General practice was not affected. Third, there were divisions between the state branches of the BMA on the question of honorary service in hospitals. Only the New South Wales and Victorian branches were strongly opposed to the payment of visiting specialists. Fourth, as mentioned above, private patients were entitled to public subsidy so that the private sector of hospital practice was perhaps as likely to expand as the public sector. Fifth, all citizens benefited from the scheme. Finally, there was no radical departure from existing practice. People were familiar with the provision of free hospital care for low-income earners. The hospital-benefits scheme simply extended this service by abolishing the means test and at the same time introducing subsidies for private patients. Thus, in the absence of unified medical opposition, the predominently Labor governments of the mid-1940s were able to implement the policy.

The hospital-benefits scheme was the only part of the proposed Commonwealth Medical Service, which came into operation during Labor's term of office. There was, however, another scheme, which was developed in cooperation with the states, namely, the anti-tuberculosis campaign. Like its hospital-benefits counterpart, this program was not the focus of medical opposition. Although the profession had objected previously to the free treatment of tuberculosis sufferers, it did not do so in the 1940s. The threat to private medical practice was minimal, especially compared with that involved in the proposal for a national medical service. There was a close connection between poverty and tuberculosis, and, because treatment involved long periods of unemployment, few sufferers could afford to pay private medical fees.

The Tuberculosis Campaign

The control of tuberculosis had long been an issue on the federal–state public-health agenda. Policy proposals had been put forward by the Federal Health Council in the late 1920s and early 1930s and by its successor, the NHMRC, but implementation had been constrained by the financial difficulties of the depression. Other factors inhibiting progress related to the problems of detection and the fact that effective treatment methods were not available until the 1940s. Under these circumstances, many of the proposals made by experts had not been implemented.

At the June 1943 health ministers' conference it was decided to embark upon an active campaign against the disease. The NHMRC was asked to outline a suitable scheme, after which the Commonwealth was to consider the extent to which financial and other assistance could be made available to the states. A second health ministers' conference in December of the same year decided to accept the NHMRC recommendations. The financial aspects were considered at the Premiers' Conference in January 1944 where it was agreed that the necessary additional facilities would be paid for on a 50–50 basis. These proposals were submitted to Cabinet with the hospital-benefits proposals, and the Tuberculosis Act was passed in 1945.[30] The Commonwealth contributed to the maintenance of diagnostic facilities, clinics, and after-care services on a 50–50 basis, up to a maximum of £50,000 per year. The hospital-benefits subsidy of six shillings per day applied to tuberculosis-hospital and sanatoria beds, as long as the states did not charge fees. In addition, a special food allowance was introduced for sufferers and their dependants in order that an appropriate diet might be taken. This latter provision was unconstitutional for the same reasons as was the 1944 Pharmaceutical Benefits Act. In 1946 the legislation was amended so that £250,000 could be paid to the states as a Section 96 grant, on the condition that the states provide the allowance (Mendelsohn 1965; Thame 1974: 85–114). Again, formal constitutional power was not necessary to achieve federal policy objectives.

In 1946, the tuberculosis division of Commonwealth Department of Health made a detailed survey of the situation in each state. Acting on the recommendations of this report, the prime minister wrote to the states in 1947, suggesting that another joint scheme be introduced. The response was positive, and a conference of federal and state officials met in April 1948, followed by a health ministers' conference in June. Negotiations were complicated by the prospect of the introduction of a national medical service that raised questions of ownership of facilities and of compensation in the event of a Commonwealth takeover. The only real disagreement concerned the proportion of new operational costs to be borne by the parties. Sir Albert Dunstan of Victoria explained that his state was 'anxious to help' but that the Commonwealth had taken all the revenue sources. The changes taking place owing to the centralization of financial power were apparent: health ministers realized that if the Commonwealth met all new expenditures, the policy-making role of the states would be very much reduced, a development about which some misgivings appeared to be emerging. The vexing question of compulsory notification was also discussed. All health ministers, except Mr White of Tasmania, agreed that compulsion was desirable, but were opposed to legislation, which they anticipated would be highly controversial. As in many other areas of health policy, Tasmania had a more advanced anti-tuberculosis program than did other states.[31]

The question of financial responsibility was resolved at the Premiers' Conference two months later. The Commonwealth agreed to bear 100 per cent of the costs of all new expenditure after 1 July 1948. The Commonwealth Tuberculosis Act received royal assent in the following November. It provided for a large-scale attack upon the disease and for more liberal financial support for sufferers. As requested, draft legislation[32] was prepared, and draft agreements were sent to the states. The federal act required that the agreements be signed by the beginning of 1950. Victoria, Queensland, Western Australia, and Tasmania complied, but South Australia and New South Wales did not. The issue of compulsion appears to have been the main problem in both states. Although agreements were made with the Commonwealth later in 1950, action on compulsion was delayed until 1952 (Mendelsohn 1965: 104–20).

An effective campaign against tuberculosis was thus launched in the early 1950s as a joint federal–state program. The Commonwealth provided the necessary additional expenditure and the broad outlines of policy. The states administered the scheme and were responsible for the coordination of new facilities and services. As with the hospital-benefits program, the cooperation of the medical profession was not essential to the introduction of the scheme. The development of an extensive anti-tuberculosis campaign proceeded steadily after 1943 in line with advances in medical science and the availability of materials and trained personnel. This process was stimulated by Tasmanian innovations in the late 1940s and was influenced by advances in New Zealand. The politics of federalism presented no substantial difficulties.

A National Medical Service

The failure of the Chifley government to implement proposals for a national medical service is not germane to this study because the major obstacles were unrelated to federalism.[33] After 1946, the Commonwealth had the necessary constitutional power. Negotiations between the national government and the national organization of the medical profession were very similar to the structure of negotiations in unitary systems of government. The following brief survey serves to illustrate the political rather than institutional nature of the obstacles.

Prior to the 1946 referendum, the federal government was aware that it lacked the necessary power to institute a national medical service. However, this did not deter policy makers from preparing plans for such a scheme. Discussions with the profession were initiated by the minister in June 1944 and were followed by a meeting of Health and Treasury officials with leaders of the BMA in the following September. At this meeting the BMA presented the following statement: 'the British Medical Association delegates are not prepared to accept a salaried medical service. Provided the Government accepts the request of the BMA Federal Council that the negotiations shall not proceed beyond the stage of discussion until one year after the war, the BMA delegates are prepared to discuss a general medical service on a fee-for-service basis.'[34]

Reporting on the meeting, the director general, Dr Cumpston, told the minister that BMA delegates thought some salaried positions might be justifiable in remote areas. In Dr Cumpston's opinion the government needed to decide whether to wait for further discussions with the profession or whether to 'determine its policy and declare that policy to the BMA and to the public.' Dr Cumpston advised that the fee-for-service system should be investigated.[35]

In anticipation of gaining the necessary constitutional power, a submission relating to Commonwealth Medical Services was put to Cabinet in November 1945. The following February, Cabinet decided that the Minister for Health should 'call a conference of State Ministers for Health to put before them proposals for a free medical service and ask for their cooperation in working out the details.'[36]

Proposals for the development of diagnostic health centres were put to a health ministers' conference in May 1946. Health minister J.M. Fraser explained to the states that this represented a stage in the provision of a complete medical service that would be available to all free of charge. Tasmania, Western Australia, and Queensland supported the proposals. New South Wales and Victoria were concerned about the effect that this expansion would have on existing services, particularly in the face of the acute shortage of nurses. New South Wales, however, supported the scheme but expressed concern about the likely attitude of the medical profession, which had already opposed a very similar state proposal. The Health minister of South Australia thought the plan desirable but was of the opinion that no action, other than planning, could be undertaken at the time because plans to expand services in his state had had to be shelved because of the lack of trained staff. As discussion proceeded, some concern was expressed about the question of ownership of existing state facilities that would need to be used as part of the new program. Finally, it was decided that a free and comprehensive medical service should be provided for all citizens and that all necessary medical centres should be established and maintained by the Commonwealth. A committee of Commonwealth and State officials was established to work on the proposals under the chairmanship of the Commonwealth director general of Health. Separate committees were set up in each state that were to include representatives of the BMA but the leaders of the profession decided not to participate.

A conference of officers was held in February 1947. Twenty-nine resolutions were adopted, which were discussed by a Health ministers' conference in May. Lengthy discussions took place about which level of government should control various aspects of the national service once it was fully developed, which would not be for some years. Various suggestions were made but, in the end, a temporary agreement was reached that the Commonwealth would develop its own central authority and provide funds and general policy direction. Administrative authority would be left with the states.[37]

In contrast with intergovernmental discussions, Commonwealth negotiations with the BMA failed to make any progress, with the result that the national medical service was not discussed at the next Health ministers' conference. In 1948, the Commonwealth made a major concession to try to break the deadlock. The National Health Service Act was passed, providing for medical benefits to be paid on a fee-for-service basis. The profession, however, remained adamantly opposed to the government scheme.[38] The legislation was a broad enabling act, providing for a national health service to be introduced by 'a process of gradual development' in agreement with the states. The establishment of health centres providing comprehensive services was authorized (CPD Senate, 24 November 1948: 3373–8; CPD HR 2 December 1948: 3929–35). In a further effort to meet objections, the legislation was amended in 1949, but no part of the scheme had come into operation when the government lost office late in the year. Negotiations with the profession had, in fact, been broken off by the government in March 1949.[39]

As had been the case with pharmaceutical benefits, members of the BMA were advised not to cooperate in any scheme that did not have the approval of the Federal Council and to refrain from responding to any approach made by the government without the approval of Branch Councils (MJA 16 April 1949: 524–5). It is interesting to speculate upon whether more might have been achieved had the Commonwealth been prepared to operate through the states by means of Section 96 grants. Three states, Tasmania, Western Australia, and New South Wales, already had small salaried medical services in rural areas, and these might have been expanded. Moreover, there was considerable support for a salaried medical service in Victoria. Both Tasmania and Queensland, and, to a lesser extent, other states, had been successful in recruiting salaried staff for their public hospitals. The states were experienced in running health services, and it seems likely that some doctors would have accepted salaried posts had the states been able to offer them. The minutes of proceedings of Health ministers' conferences show that there was little opposition to an expansion of services along the lines suggested by the JCSS and the NHMRC. With the necessary financial resources, state governments might have been able to expand some of their existing services, and even introduce new ones. In retrospect, it seems that there was not the slightest chance that the Commonwealth could negotiate an agreement with the BMA on the introduction of a national health service, even on a part-time or fee-for-service basis.

Conclusion

The 1940s were characterized by a high level of cooperation between State and Commonwealth policy makers. This experience shows that cooperative federalism can be a reality under certain conditions and that the processes of joint decision making do not necessarily lead to obstruction and delay. Cooperation in the 1940s was facilitated by the fact that Labor governments were in power in most jurisdictions, which gave rise to broad agreement on the main outlines, if not the details, of policy proposals.

Although the Curtin and Chifley governments took the view that health should be a function of the Commonwealth, and, in this, they were generally supported by members of state Labor governments, the evidence shows that the centralization of power was not essential to policy implementation. The hospital-benefits scheme, which was, in fact, a set of financial arrangements, was introduced in cooperation with the states. The eradication of tuberculosis was a public-health program, and, in this sphere, a pattern of intergovernmental cooperation had been in place since the 1920s. It appears to have been assumed, however, that the two new programs, the national medical service and the pharmaceutical-benefits scheme, should be exclusively Commonwealth functions. Health minister N.E. McKenna acknowledged in 1947 that the pharmaceutical-benefits scheme should have been allowed to develop gradually, along with the expansion of other services. Such development could have been achieved from the outset by the provision of free medicines through existing state institutions, particularly in the outpatients departments of public hospitals. As Canadian and other Australian policy experience shows, the power to provide financial assistance to state and provincial governments is a useful and important instrument of policy promotion that can be used in the absence of formal constitutional power. When the decision in the first *Pharmaceutical Benefits* case indicated that the Commonwealth did not have the power to pay the proposed special allowance to tuberculosis sufferers, the legislation was amended and the money was directed through the states by means of Section 96 grants. This method of policy development might have been used in other areas, allowing the states to expand their services as wartime shortages were overcome. Labor's traditional attitude towards federalism appears to have been the main reason that this approach was not taken.

Australian experience, then, like its Canadian counterpart, demonstrates that federalism is not a safeguard against the development and implementation of radical policies. The federal division of power did not prevent policies developed in some jurisdictions from becoming national in scope. The initiatives taken in Queensland and Tasmania earlier in the century culminated in the introduction of a national system of universally available free hospital care in the 1940s. As in Canada, reform proposals emerged at different times at both levels of government. The plan for a national health service was very similar to the proposals developed in New South Wales between 1910 and 1916. The links between earlier state initiatives and Commonwealth policy of the 1940s are less direct than the links between provincial health-insurance plans and federal-government policy in Canada but, in general, the plan for a national health service was an extension and expansion of policies and ideas that had previously developed in the more innovative states.

The development of Australian health policy up to the 1940s therefore lends considerable support to the 'revisionist' theory of federalism. However, after this time the centralization of constitutional and financial power and the activist role taken by federal governments of both political persuasions severely limited the capacity of the states to pursue independent policy lines. In the health area, at least, the 'revisionist' theory lost most of its usefulness in explaining the dynamics of Australian federalism.

The orthodox idea that federalism allows interest groups undue influence in policy processes is not supported by the evidence from the 1940s. The profession was not able to obstruct the introduction of free hospital care, a policy in which both levels of government were involved, but it was able to completely defeat the two new Commonwealth initiatives. In both Canada and Australia, experience suggests that support of opposition parties, which, of course, reflects perceptions of public opinion, is crucial to the success of the medical profession in defeating government proposals. The BMA was defeated in Tasmania when both Labor and non-Labor governments pursued similar policies between 1914 and 1923. In contrast, the opposition in New South Wales supported the doctors' stand between 1910 and 1916 when the Labor government was able to achieve only some of its aims. And, in the 1940s, the opposition parties and the profession campaigned actively against Labor's collectivist policies. In the absence of strong public support, such as existed in Saskatchewan and Quebec, the BMA was able to persist in its refusal to cooperate with the government. Under these circumstances, the constitutional protection offered by the clause prohibiting civil conscription was of little practical significance.

Although Australia is a federal system, in many respects its health-policy development followed a parallel course with Britain's and New Zealand's. In these countries, governments increasingly assumed responsibility for the provision of hospital and other health services from the nineteenth century onwards. Policy developed less evenly in Australia because of federal arrangements but, in some jurisdictions, notably in Queensland and Tasmania, government responsibility for hospital services preceded similar developments in Britain. The main difference in this area between Australia and Britain was that the British government became involved in the subsidization of a limited system of health insurance in 1911, whereas Australian governments did not. However, as we will see in the next chapter, Australia attempted to follow British practice in this area as well. The proposals failed, not because of institutional arrangements, but because the Australian medical profession was far more united than its British counterpart in its opposition to insurance. Developments in the two countries culminated in the 1940s in sets of proposals that were very similar in principle, if not in detail, showing that ideas and traditions were a more important determinant of policy than were institutional arrangements.

At first sight it may appear that the governments of unitary Britain and New Zealand were more successful in achieving their health-policy objectives in the 1940s than was the federal government in Australia. Even if this were so, it would need be shown that obstacles and delays emanated from federal arrangements rather than from other factors in order to establish that federalism retards policy development. However, closer inspection shows that both the British and the New Zealand governments were only partly successful in achieving their objectives. In New Zealand, doctors were not united but, even so, the government was forced to introduce fee-for-service in 1941 after two and a half years of physician non-cooperation. It had little control of either medical services or the pharmaceutical-benefits system. Australian policy makers considered that abuses were rampant and that services to patients were poor so that, in several respects, the New Zealand 'system' served as an example of what not to do.

In Britain, the medical profession was also divided. There had long been antipathy and competition between specialists and general practitioners, a situation that was partly based upon class distinctions. Moreover, there was a radical group within the profession that strongly supported the development of a salaried medical service. The introduction of the National Health Service in 1948 was not a radical policy formulated by a socialist Labor government. It was, rather, an extension to the whole country of a system that had developed in large city hospitals where consultants had been successful in excluding general practitioners from hospital practice. As Abel-Smith (1979: xvi) has argued, it was what the leaders of the medical profession, the specialists, wanted.

Despite the sovereignty of Parliament and the deep divisions within the medical profession, the British government, like the Australian, failed in its efforts to introduce a salaried-general-practitioner medical service. The deadlock between the BMA and the Minister for Health, Aneurin Bevan, was broken only when Bevan agreed to exclude the possibility of a salaried service. In Britain's version of Australia's constitutional clause prohibiting the civil conscription of doctors and dentists, the 1949 act amending the National Health Service Act incorporated a statutory ban on salaried service for general practice (Blanpain 1978: 216). Because Bevan hoped that the profession would eventually accept a salaried service, this was the concession he had been most eager to avoid (Honigsbaum 1979: 284–98). The governments of the 1940s in unitary Britain and New Zealand and in federal Australia failed to achieve all of their health-policy objectives because they could not gain the cooperation of the medical profession.

4

Voluntary Health Insurance in Australia, 1950–72

In December 1949, the federal Labor government, which had attempted to introduce a national health service, was replaced by a Liberal–Country party coalition government with very different aims. Non-Labor favoured a policy of minimum government intervention in welfare areas. It opposed the public provision of services, which it thought undermined thrift and self-reliance and led to excessive dependence upon government. Where intervention was necessary to supplement a market distribution of resources, as in the case of income support for the aged, non-Labor favoured contributory systems of social insurance. Tax-based methods of financing social policies were opposed because of the burden such systems placed on the treasury.

The Menzies federal government introduced its own national health scheme between 1950 and 1953. This publicly subsidized system of voluntary health insurance was very different from the national health service proposed by Labor in the 1940s. It met non-Labor's objectives and had been formulated by the medical profession. The BMA in Australia had opposed health insurance since its introduction in Britain in 1911. It was not until the 1940s that a private insurance system that would include middle-income earners was devised and promoted by the BMA. However, fee-for-service insurance is expensive, and attempts to develop profession-sponsored plans were not successful until the willingness of non-Labor to provide a public subsidy made private insurance a viable proposition.

Voluntary health insurance changed the course of Australian health-policy development. The long trend towards the public provision of services was reversed, and private medical practice became firmly entrenched. The replacement of friendly-society contract practice resulted in substantial income gains for doctors at the cost of more expensive insurance premiums for citizens.

A second important effect of Commonwealth health policy was a substantial reduction of the role of the states both in relation to the public hospitals that they administered and with respect to overall policy development. Whereas the states had been responsible for expanding service provision and for supervising contract practice, after 1950 their capacity to contribute to policy was reduced and their stance became almost entirely reactive. To create a demand for private insurance, it was necessary to abolish Labor's system of free hospital care. The financial dominance of the Commonwealth and its constitutional power to frame its health benefits in support of the health-care delivery system that it favoured were sufficient to compel all states except Queensland to comply. On the hospital side, non-Labor policy deliberately promoted the independence of hospitals and the independence of doctors working in them by reducing reliance on direct government funds. Over time, a failure to increase benefit levels led to a considerable drop in the Commonwealth's share of hospital operating costs, so that the states were faced with the difficult choice of instituting politically unpopular fee increases or of finding alternative sources of revenue. Responsibility for service provision remained with the states by default but, by the late 1960s, their financial capacity to offer a comprehensive range of services was severely curtailed.

Much of the Commonwealth's dominant position arose from the financial powers it acquired during the Second World War, but the constitutional referendum of 1946 is also important. Prior to the 1940s, there was no clear definition of the Commonwealth's power in relation to social insurance. However, the 1946 referendum established without question the Commonwealth's power in relation to health services and benefits. The non-Labor government elected in 1949 inherited an amplitude of constitutional and financial power that enabled it to establish a system that remained virtually unchanged despite widespread criticism during its twenty-three-year tenure of office.

Health Insurance and the Medical Profession

The main purpose of the political activity of the medical profession in Australia (and in most similar countries) has been to preserve the size of the private medical market. In the private market, there is no intermediary between the patient and the doctor. The patient pays a fee for each service, the level of which is determined by the doctor. Before the advent of public subsidization, many people could not afford to pay private fees. Under these circumstances, mutual aid societies, known variously as friendly societies, clubs, or lodges, came to provide a means of access to medical services. Members paid a small weekly sum to a society, which contracted with doctors to provide services. Doctors were paid an annual capitation fee for each person who was entitled to treatment, irrespective of the number of services actually provided. In Britain, society member-ship covered only the contributor but, in Australia, a member's family was also covered. Doctors always objected to this form of practice and, in Australia, fought hard and successfully to limit its expansion.[1]

For twenty-five years after national health insurance was introduced in Britain in 1911, the Australian medical profession vehemently opposed the scheme. British doctors had gained financially from insurance, but this did not make the system attractive to Australian doctors.[2] An editorial in the *Australasian Medical Gazette* in 1913 voiced the official view: 'we reiterate what we have said on previous occasions, that, quite apart from any ques-tion of remuneration or probable diminution in the amount of fees to be earned by medical men, the wholesale conversion of private into contract practice ... must inevitably lead to a deterioration in the calibre of the medical man, to the lowering of the standard of work ... and increased suffering on the part of the sick' (24 May 1913: 490). The leaders of the profession in Australia equated contract practice with 'slavery.'

Before the 1930s, the stance of the profession was entirely defensive. It insisted that there was no pauper class in Australia and that there was thus no need for insurance. It opposed the expansion of directly pro-vided services and of the public hospital system and succeeded in limit-ing friendly-society membership to low-income earners. Asked by the Royal Commission on National Insurance in 1923 to formulate princi-ples for a national insurance scheme, the Federal Committee of the BMA told the commission that 'no existing form of national health insurance would be acceptable' (*MJA* 2 May 1925: 457; 2 August 1924: 125–31). Doc-tors were instrumental in having a separate royal commission on health appointed in 1925. The commission was chaired by the president of the Federal Committee, and another two of the five commissioners were prominent members of the association. The report recommended an ex-pansion of public-health services through federal-state cooperation[3] and avoided the question of insurance altogether.

Depression conditions and a fear of 'nationalization' led to the devel-opment of a more positive approach in the 1930s. The Queensland Branch put forward a proposal for a Complete Medical Service based on the

British system of insurance in 1934. There was to be no income limit, and general practitioners were to be paid on a capitation basis.[4] Queensland doctors feared that their government had 'in mind the establishment of a widespread medical service' with free treatment for everyone.[5] When proposals for national insurance re-emerged at the federal level in the mid-1930s, the Federal Council gave its approval to a scheme that was similar to the British system. However, the details of this scheme were not well worked out (Thame 1974: 308–10).

In the face of the Labor government's proposals in the 1940s, the need to formulate a policy that would extend access to services for middle-income groups but preserve a large private medical market became urgent. Opinion within the branches and within the Federal Council was divided. At this time, private practice was less extensive than has often been assumed. Although the extent of contract practice had been reduced, friendly societies still provided medical services for 29 per cent of the population in 1938 (Green and Cromwell 1984: 130–40, 221). Under contract practice, doctors were employed by the societies on contract and were paid on the basis of a capitation fee for each patient for whom they were responsible. In addition, about 18 per cent of the population received medical services in the outpatients' departments of public hospitals, a trend that was expanding.[6] There were also a number of industry-based schemes where doctors were engaged on contract or salary, and salaried services had been established in rural areas of three states. The war led to an extension of non-private medical practice in the forces, munitions factories, and repatriation establishments. Moreover, within the private medical sector there were many people who could not afford fees and were treated free or at a reduced rate. In the hospital sector, most services were provided on an honorary or salaried basis.[7] Thus private practice had not been established as the only, or even the dominant, mode of practice in the 1940s. The situation in Australia shared similarities with that in Britain before public subsidization was introduced. As Klein (1977: 164) has recorded, 'the golden age of professional practice existed only for some doctors. In reality the medical proletariat – scraping a precarious income without any sort of financial safety net – were rescued first by the introduction of national insurance in 1911 and then by the creation of the National Health Service.'

The challenge for the Australian profession was to develop a policy that would enable people to pay for services without bringing about an extension of contract practice or salaried service (*MJA* 1 November 1941: 513, 521; 24 April 1943: 371–8; 28 October 1944: 460–8).

Gradually support began to emerge for a system of private insurance for middle-income earners in which patients would pay doctors on a fee-for-service basis. As in the case of opposition to national insurance in 1938 (see below), the New South Wales branch took the lead in policy development. In 1946, one thousand doctors subscribed £10 each in order to establish a medical-benefits fund. Later, a similar scheme was started in Victoria, but, in the absence of government subsidy, expansion was slow (Sax 1984: 59–60). However, the profession had at last found an insurance system that met its objectives. In 1949, BMA policy was published in a booklet, entitled *A National Health Service.*[8] For the middle-income group, voluntary insurance schemes based on the Medical Benefits Fund of New South Wales were to be set up. For the lower-income group, the existing system of contract practice was to continue and the government was to pay for a general-practitioner service for pensioners and the unemployed. Any additional assistance that governments wished to provide should be paid directly to patients, the Federal Council argued (BMA 1949: 12–13). While these proposals were unacceptable to the Labor party, they were in accordance with non-Labor's approach to the provision of social services.

Non-Labor and the Principle of Insurance

The approach of the non-Labor parties to health insurance was influenced, historically, by their preferred method of financing other social policies, particularly old-age pensions, which have always been funded from general revenue in Australia. Interest in contributory insurance was stimulated by the passage of the Lloyd George Act of 1911 in Britain. Both the Liberal and the Labor parties considered the contributory system at this time but, whereas it found support within the Liberal party, it was rejected by Labor. At the National Conference of the Labor party in 1912, the view was put forward that 'a system of contributory insurance is not a sound one. Such insurance should be a direct charge on the community and not on portion of the worker's wages.'[9]

Contributory insurance was part of the Liberal platform in the 1913 election campaign but the party gained office with only a narrow majority and did not attempt to introduce legislation. No action was taken during the war or in the reconstruction period but, in 1923, the Nationalist–Country party government appointed a royal commission to inquire into national insurance. The government argued that social services should be 'placed on a satisfactory and permanent basis to remove altogether the taint of pauperism' (quoted in Kewley 1973: 143). In 1928, a national insurance bill was introduced into Parliament. The bill made provision for widows' and orphans' benefits as well as for sickness, invalidity, and old age, but did not include health insurance. However, it soon became apparent that there was little support for the scheme and, in the face of opposition from employers, insurance companies, and the friendly societies, the legislation was abandoned (Kewley 1973: 143–9; Watts 1983: 88–92).

In the search for a means of reducing government expenditure during the depression, the old-age-pension system came under intense scrutiny. The idea that the tax-based method of financing pensions had been a 'mistake' became the dominant view among liberal reformers and financial conservatives alike (Watts 1983: 93–120). When legislation finally emerged in 1938, health insurance was included largely because Sir Walter Kinnear, who had been brought from England to prepare a report, considered that health and pensions schemes 'should be treated as one organic whole.'[10]

The 1938 proposals drew criticism from a wide range of groups, including the medical profession, the friendly societies, the Labor party, the Communist party, and some members of both parties in the governing coalition.[11] Although opinion was divided, medical opposition was the main reason that the proposals were finally abandoned (Sax 1984: 41–2; Watts 1983: 161–219).

Debates on the legislation revealed the wide differences that had developed between Labor and non-Labor concerning methods of financing social services. Treasurer R.G. Casey, moving the second reading of the bill, argued that 'in view of the impending liability of the existing pensions scheme ... I say quite frankly that unless something is done to put these schemes on a contributory basis, no government of the future ... could embark upon any worthwhile extension of our social services without seriously threatening the whole financial fabric of the Commonwealth' (quoted in Kewley 1973: 159). In contrast, Opposition leader John Curtin expressed the Labor position: 'the Labor Party expresses its utter condemnation of individual contributions as a principle in regard to invalidity, old-age and widow's pensions. These services should be a charge upon the consolidated revenue of the Commonwealth ... The Labor Party believes that the time has arrived when national health services should be treated, in principle, in the same way as education. They should be free to all members of the community' (quoted in Kewley 1973: 162).

Both 1938 proposals and the taxation arrangements for social services introduced by Labor in the 1940s involved the taxation of people whose incomes had previously fallen below the tax threshold. However, Labor's policies maintained the principle of income-related taxation. Flat-rate individual contributions were rejected entirely. As Kewley has argued, 'the 1945 arrangements, in essence, merely provided for the older, as well as the newer social services to be financed indirectly, instead of directly from the Consolidated Revenue Fund' (1973: 245). In contrast, non-Labor policy was intended to minimize general-revenue financing as far as possible. The voluntary health-insurance system proposed by the BMA achieved this objective. It was also in accordance with non-Labor arguments that the contributory principle preserved self-respect, encouraged thrift, and eliminated the idea of 'handouts.'

The Implementation of BMA Policy

In December 1949, Sir Earle Page, former surgeon, former treasurer and deputy prime minister, and advocate of contributory insurance in 1928 and again in 1938, became minister for Health. A month later, with Cabinet authorization, he began negotiations with the BMA, the friendly societies, and the Pharmaceutical Guild. In the meantime, the Federal Council of the BMA had met to formulate a set of proposals for the minister. It was resolved that the 'hospital problem' should be given first priority through the reimposition of the means test and increased government financing. The profession decided that it was willing to participate in the free provision of a limited range of costly medicines and that the federal government should be asked to subsidize voluntary hospital insurance and a medical service for pensioners on a fee-for-service basis. No resolution was passed concerning general medical benefits, indicating that there was still uncertainty about government intervention in this area. When the minister met with the council, he was told that the profession would not cooperate in any scheme that involved government control. A joint meeting was then held with members of the BMA and the friendly societies, and the minister held discussions with the executive of the Pharmaceutical Guild.[12]

In January 1950 a submission was presented to Cabinet. The proposals were those that had been 'recommended and agreed by the various organisations.' Arrangements for medical benefits were those set out by the BMA in 1949: a capitation system for low-income earners and voluntary insurance for higher-income earners with doctors paid on a fee-for-service basis. It was argued that the subsidization of voluntary effort avoided many of the pitfalls of universal compulsory schemes and that the scheme gave the treasury 'definite control' of expenditures.[13] A committee of four ministers was authorized to prepare a detailed submission for consideration, which was presented to Cabinet in April. The adoption of voluntary insurance was strongly recommended. Evidence from the United States was presented in support of the recommendations.[14]

At this time, however, the New South Wales branch of the BMA changed its policy. On 1 April 1950, it decided that all contract practice with friendly societies should be abolished. In discussions with the minister, the president of the Federal Council said that, as far as he was aware, there was no similar movement in Victoria. The possibility of replacing contract practice with a new system of fee-for-service based on concessional rates was discussed. The minister argued that the proposed BMA fee of 9/6 per consultation should be reduced to 7/6 since the return under contract at the time amounted to only 4/9 per service. Because only the New South Wales branch had rejected contract practice, no decision on the matter was made.[15]

After further discussions with the BMA, the minister met with the federal executive of the friendly societies. He said that the government would not become involved in the question of whether contract practice should continue. If it survived, it would be subsidized. Otherwise, it would be replaced by fee-for-service on a concessional basis for members of friendly societies.[16]

The following month, the BMA abandoned its support for contract practice for low-income earners (Green and Cromwell 1984: 169). Later in the year, the New South Wales branch circularized its members as follows:

you are warned that should the profession in this State decide to continue Friendly Society practice on a Capitation Fee basis ... the Health Service policy of the Association will almost certainly be defeated. Should we at this late stage endorse a capitation rate Friendly Society service, which would be easy to administer if put on a national basis, we cannot expect any government to grant our request for a Fee for Service system which will be so much more difficult to administer. It is therefore the opinion of this Federation that all practitioners should terminate the current Common Form of Agreement before a National Health Scheme is introduced.' (quoted in Green and Cromwell 1984: 168)

When the medical-benefits scheme was introduced in July 1953, contract practice had been abolished, except in a few isolated instances. The minister had not been able to achieve a concessional rate for members of friendly societies. A full fee-for-service was charged, increasing the doctors' return per consultation from 4/9 to 12/6, with a commensurate increase in the cost of the insurance premiums paid by the community.

The elimination of contract practice is important for several reasons. First, it is not commonly known that payment by capitation was to have been part of the Earle Page scheme.[17] It is by using financial incentives and regulations under the contract system that British governments have been able to influence the distribution of services. Second, the introduction of fee-for-service at a non-concessional rate demonstrates the extent to which the Menzies government was prepared to allow the BMA to dictate policy. The government was in a strong position to bargain in relation to subsidization rates and in relation to the details, if not the principles, of the scheme. In terms of financial arrangements, the profession's interests were put before those of contributors. Finally, and most importantly, while centralization facilitated the adoption of a uniform system of medical benefits in all states, it was a system based on the preferences of the most militant branch of the profession in the country. If responsibility for health policy had remained decentralized, it is safe to assume that policy outcomes in some states would have reflected the less radical position of branches of the BMA outside New South Wales. As we will see below, state governments were eager to ensure that payment by the fee-for-service method in hospitals should not be extended. However, the states were not involved in policy making in relation to medical services in the early 1950s.

In other important respects, the Earle Page system was based on the BMA's preferences. The pharmaceutical-benefits scheme, introduced in September 1950, provided for only a limited number of free medicines, amounting to 20 per cent of prescriptions.[18] The pensioner medical service, which began in 1951, was the scheme proposed by the profession in 1949. Services were limited to those provided by general practitioners, as the BMA had suggested. The only part of the 1949 BMA policy that the government did not introduce was a set of special arrangements for the unemployed.

The federal government had the constitutional power it needed to introduce medical- and pharmaceutical-benefits schemes and a pensioner medical service without reference to the states. In addition, it had the financial power to induce all states, except Queensland, to comply with BMA policy in relation to the 'hospital problem.'

The Termination of Labor's Free Hospital Scheme

Proposals for a new hospital-benefits scheme were put to Cabinet in April

1950. The stated objectives were to enable people to obtain insurance at low cost, to restore 'full control and unfettered administration of hospitals to hospital management,' and to provide a substantial portion of the costs of hospital maintenance from non-government sources. A flat-rate subsidy was to be paid to members of approved voluntary insurance organizations, who were to pay flat-rate premiums. The government subsidy and the fund benefits were to be used by members to pay hospital costs. Administration of the scheme was to be the responsibility of the funds, and administrative costs were to be met from contributions. Hospitals were to be permitted to reintroduce fees in public wards. Cabinet approved, in principle, of the recommendations.[19]

The scheme was discussed at a Health ministers' conference in August 1950 and was not enthusiastically received. Hospital costs had been rising rapidly, and state ministers unanimously requested an increase in federal subsidies. Both the Queensland and Tasmanian ministers (Labor) were strongly opposed to any alteration of the existing scheme. New South Wales (Labor) opposed a reintroduction of the means test, and the Victorian minister (Country party) suggested that compulsory insurance should be considered. Sir Earle Page rejected the latter proposal, which he said would 'result in governmental control of the whole show.' No decisions were reached other than that requirements for new hospital facilities should be studied. The Commonwealth made it clear that its share of hospital funding would not be increased, a strategy that put pressure on the states to accept the new scheme.[20]

A second federal-state conference was held in January 1951. The Commonwealth announced that it intended to terminate the existing hospital agreements when they expired the following year. The 1950 proposals were again put to the states except that the subsidy for insured patients was to be increased from 9/- to 12/-. The federal government offered to meet the cost of medicines used in public hospitals in those states with which new agreements were negotiated.

All states except Western Australia (Liberal–Country party) remained opposed to the reintroduction of charges. The general view put forward was that people were paying a social-security tax and had been told that governments would finance hospitals. Victoria insisted that it was a Commonwealth responsibility to raise any extra taxes that were necessary because it now dominated the taxation field. The very strong financial position of the Commonwealth was discussed. The Western Australian minister thought that voluntary insurance would probably work but said that, if it did not, the scheme could be placed on a compulsory basis. New

South Wales and Victoria favoured compulsory insurance, and Tasmania indicated interest, but Sir Earle Page said that such a scheme was tantamount to 'nationalization.'[21] He again stated clearly that there would be no increase in federal financial assistance, except through the system devised by the Commonwealth.

After lengthy discussion, it was resolved that those sections of the existing agreements to which the federal government objected would be removed, including the section that prohibited fee-charging in public wards of hospitals. The Commonwealth would meet the cost of life-saving drugs for public-hospital patients, and the existing subsidy would continue to be paid. The states would not be forced to reimpose a means test, and the introduction of arrangements to promote voluntary insurance would be at the discretion of individual states. The resolutions amounted to a partial defeat for the Commonwealth.[22]

After the conference, bilateral negotiations took place. An agreement that met with Commonwealth requirements was reached with Western Australia, and a copy of the draft agreement was circulated to other states. Negotiations proceeded satisfactorily with South Australia (Liberal) but were delayed because of the special circumstances of country hospitals, which were partly funded from local-government taxation. The Victorian political situation was complex. A minority Country party government held office with Labor party support. It asked the Commonwealth to postpone negotiations until the following year. Queensland was willing to enter into a new agreement but only on the condition that free treatment in public hospitals be continued. Negotiations with Tasmania failed to reach agreement, and New South Wales refused to declare its position on the issue.[23]

When the hospital agreements expired on 20 August 1952, the Commonwealth broke the undertaking that Sir Earle Page had given at the 1951 Health ministers' conference. The states were informed that the federal subsidy was no longer payable, except to insured patients through insurance organizations. The response was swift. A week later, the Tasmanian premier sent a telegram 'approving in principle of an agreement on the Commonwealth Government's Hospital scheme.' On 10 September, New South Wales announced that a new federal–state hospital agreement would operate from 1 October, from which time public patients would be charged fees. Agreements were finalized with South Australia. In Victoria, the decision to comply with the Commonwealth's terms resulted in the defeat of the government. At the ensuing election, Labor was elected to office and a week later accepted the scheme it had voted

against to defeat the previous government. Inglis (1958: 199) argues that
'Labor was equally impotent in the face of the Commonwealth government's determination to make grants for hospitals only to states accepting its scheme.' While this assessment is valid, it perhaps overestimates
the importance of financial factors and underestimates the force of political
considerations. Victoria, as the second-largest state, was essential to the
success of the Commonwealth scheme and thus might have had a stronger
bargaining position than Queensland. The different positions taken by
the two Labor governments reflect the very different historical approaches
to health policy in the two states. Whereas considerable support for voluntarism remained in Victoria, access to hospitals had long been considered a right in Queensland.[24]

In contrast with its counterpart in Victoria, the Queensland government remained adamant that 'free' hospital treatment would continue.
After a series of letters between the premier and the prime minister, a
compromise was reached that was influenced by the forthcoming Senate
and state government elections. In October 1952, the prime minister accepted Queensland's offer 'to provide non-public ward hospital accommodation' as a basis for a new agreement. Thus Queensland continued
to receive the existing Commonwealth subsidy without introducing either public-ward hospital charges or a means test.[25] Tasmania was later
to complain that the agreement made with Queensland was based on an
undertaking that arrangements satisfactory to the Commonwealth would
be made in the future, whereas the agreements with other states were
concluded only after such arrangements had already been made. In 1953
and again in 1955, Tasmania attempted to negotiate new terms and conditions with the Commonwealth but was unsuccessful on both occasions.[26]

Federalism did frustrate the Commonwealth's aims in relation to hospital policy in Queensland. But in all other states and in all other aspects
of the national health scheme, the constitutional and financial power of
the federal government was sufficient to enable the full implementation
of its policies.

The Impact of Centralization on State Hospitals

Commonwealth policy had a significant impact on the hospital sector. As
discussed in chapter 3, even the least interventionist states had taken steps
to control hospital policy in the years prior to the Second World War. The
Menzies government and the medical profession wanted to reverse this
trend. Commonwealth benefits for the insured were channelled not through

TABLE 3
All general hospitals – sources of revenue

Year	Commonwealth	State	Total public	Insurance	Net fees	Total private
1960–61	30	43	73	13	14	27
1963–64	31	41	72	17	11	28
1966–67	28	41	69	21	10	31
1969–70	21	49	70	21	9	30
1972–73	16	50	66	22	13	34
1974–75	13	55	67	26	7	33

SOURCES: Deeble (1970: 121; 1982a: 719)

the states but through insurance funds to individual patients. The uninsured benefit, which was not increased between 1947 and 1970, was paid to the states until 1962. However, on the expiration of the hospital agreements in that year, this benefit, along with the pensioner benefit and a new federal nursing-home benefit, became payable directly to hospitals. As Sax has argued, 'the effect ... was to eliminate direct assistance to the states for the operation of public hospitals and most nursing homes while emphasising commonwealth assistance to individuals to help them meet the costs of their care. Of course, the states derived benefit indirectly ... [but] the cost to the states of this type of assistance was the curtailment of their capacity to plan a rational distribution of health services' (1984: 73).

Commonwealth policy not only undermined the states' control of hospitals but it also increased their share of financial responsibility. In the 1960s and early 1970s, the proportion of hospital-maintenance costs borne by the federal government steadily declined while the states' share steadily increased. Table 3 shows these trends.

The percentage of hospital revenue met by the Commonwealth fell from 31 per cent in 1963–4 to 13 per cent in 1974–5 whereas the state share increased from 41 to 55 per cent during the same period. This change in the balance of financial responsibility was achieved in a relatively invisible way: both the insured and the uninsured benefits were held static, which caused their real value to fall dramatically. The share of Commonwealth funding would have fallen by more had fewer citizens taken private insurance. The prospect of having to pay large hospital bills was sufficient to ensure that most people held at least some level of insurance coverage, so that the real value of the subsidy did not need to be maintained.

In summary, the voluntary health insurance system met most of the objectives of the non-Labor government and the medical profession. For the government's part, at least one major social policy was placed on a contributory basis. Responsibility for administration was contracted out to voluntary organizations, and the community met the administrative costs. The Commonwealth was able to control its share of expenditure. In fact, there was no commitment to meet or maintain any specified proportion of the costs of either hospital or medical services. The proportion of costs reimbursed to patients depended on the fees charged by the hospital, the means test that was applied, and the level of insurance coverage held. For medical services, reimbursement levels depended on the fee charged by the doctor. Thus, it was not obvious if the value of the Commonwealth subsidy fell.

For the medical profession, the financial viability of private practice was established, and the long battle to eliminate contract practice was finally won. The reimbursement system meant that there was no intermediary between the doctor and the patient, except in the case of the pensioner medical service. Patients were free to choose their doctors, and doctors their patients.[27] There was no federal intervention in the organization of the health-care system such as had been planned in the 1940s. Doctors were free to decide what services would be provided, where practices would be located, and what fees would be charged. The capacity of the states to provide alternative and supplementary services was limited by their general financial dependency and their increasing indebtedness (Mathews and Jay 1972: 196–7; Whitlam 1971: 8). Thus, the threat to the size of the private medical market that directly provided services had presented in the first half of the century was largely removed. Although the system met the objectives of its sponsors, by the 1960s it had become a political liability.

Rising Criticism of the Voluntary Health-Insurance System

During the second half of the 1960s, most aspects of Australian social policy came under scrutiny. It was discovered that, although there had been many years of economic prosperity, some citizens had failed to benefit and that pockets of serious poverty existed (Kewley 1973: 391–3). Social-security benefits were said to be so inadequate that they gave rise to poverty instead of providing a defence against it (Tierney 1970: 217–18). Australia was one of the few OECD countries in which the proportion of

GDP spent on income maintenance fell during the 1960s (Sheehan 1980: 115).

One of the most controversial aspects of social policy was the health-insurance system. Dissatisfaction first arose in the late 1950s because reimbursement rates had fallen as medical fees had risen.[28] In response to criticism, the federal government increased its subsidy in 1960. However, the benefit was not passed on to patients because doctors immediately raised their fees. Thereafter, governments were reluctant to increase subsidies unless the AMA[29] could give an assurance that fee increases would be controlled. The AMA, however, had no power to offer such assurance and could only make recommendations to members.

By the late 1960s, criticism of the system reached the proportions of a national debate. Controversy was fuelled by the research findings of two economists, R.B. Scotton and J.S. Deeble. According to Kewley, their work was largely responsible for the informed nature of the criticism, which was difficult for the government to dismiss (Kewley 1973: 391). In 1968, the Labor party succeeded in securing the appointment of a Senate select committee to examine hospital and medical costs and other aspects of the health-care system. Two weeks later, the government responded by appointing an independent committee of inquiry into health insurance. The committee's terms of reference, however, were narrow. Sixteen specific questions were to be investigated, and the committee was invited to make such other recommendations as it deemed necessary 'within the context of the voluntary health insurance system.'

The committee's report was presented in March 1969 (Nimmo Report).[30] In the course of its investigations, the committee studied arrangements in other countries and three members visited Canada to look at the way responsibility for financing health policy was shared between levels of government. Several of the 'lessons to be drawn from Canada's experience' were incorporated in the recommendations (Nimmo Report 1969: 67–70).

In relation to the Australian system, the committee 'endorsed practically all of the criticisms which had been levelled at the scheme, especially those of Scotton and Deeble' (Kewley 1969: 504). Its findings were as follows:

1 The operation of the health insurance scheme is unnecessarily complex and beyond the comprehension of many.
2 The benefits received by contributors are frequently much less than the cost of hospital and medical services.

3 The contributions have increased to such an extent that they are beyond the capacity of some members of the community and involve considerable hardship for others.
4 The rules of many registered organisations including the so-called 'special account' rules permit disallowance or reduction of claims for particular conditions. The application of these rules causes serious and widespread hardship.
5 An unduly high proportion of the contributions received by some organisations is absorbed by operating expenses.
6 The level of reserves held by some organisations is unnecessarily high. (Nimmo Report 1969: 9)

It was also noted that, because hospital and medical fees were unpredictable, funds could not guarantee adequate protection to members. Some funds had engaged in 'excessive self promotion' and had paid 'insufficient attention to the "non-profit" nature of the scheme'[31] (Nimmo Report 1969: 15).

The committee's recommendations were that a national health-insurance commission be established, that benefit tables be simplified, that low-income families be assisted with premium payments, that subsidies for the chronically ill be increased, and that the funds be placed under greater regulation and control. In relation to hospital access, the committee recommended that standard ward accommodation 'be available to every member of the community regardless of means.' It was argued that patients should be free to choose intermediate or private accommodation rather than being forced to accept more expensive accommodation on the basis of a means test. The system proposed was similar to that operating in Tasmania, where there were few non-public hospital wards. The honorary system was to be gradually abolished.

The method of stabilizing medical benefits that the committee recommended was borrowed directly from Canada. A medical-benefits schedule based on 'the most common fee' was to be introduced. It was argued that schedules had operated in Canada for many years with good results. Further, it was recommended that a participating-doctor scheme, which had operated in Canadian profession-sponsored insurance plans, should be introduced. Other proposals drawn from Canadian experience included special arrangements for low-income earners, methods of premium collection, administrative arrangements, and methods of federal–state cost-sharing. Of these recommendations only three were implemented at the time. The others formed part of the compulsory scheme introduced in 1975, with the exception of the proposal for a participating-doctor scheme, which no Australian government has so far attempted to introduce. The influence of Canadian experience is a clear example of the 'demonstration effect' created by successful policies and of the way ideas frequently spread from country to country.

The question of equity was outside the committee's terms of reference but the scheme had also been criticized on these grounds. The combination of flat-rate premiums and the tax deductibility of patient co-payments and premiums meant that both insurance and the patient share of health-care costs became cheaper as income increased. The erosion of the real value of the Commonwealth hospital benefit, together with hospital-fee policy, had the effect of increasing the proportionate cost of public-ward care. By 1967, it was calculated that it was cheaper for a person earning four times average weekly earnings to buy family insurance for private-ward coverage than it was for a person earning 75 per cent of average weekly earnings (who qualified by income) to buy family insurance for public-ward coverage (Scotton 1978; Deeble 1970: 68–73, 272–3).

While the Nimmo Committee had been conducting its investigations, the Labor party had adopted proposals for a universal health-insurance scheme. The insurance debate then shifted from the problems of the existing system to a discussion of the merits of voluntary insurance compared with those of a compulsory system. The pressure on the government to take decisive action was thereby increased, particularly since 1969 was an election year.

Reform of the Voluntary Health-Insurance System

The Liberal–Country party government in the late 1960s was led by an assertive and centralist prime minister, John Gorton, who was 'not averse to preempting Labor's proposals' (Sax 1984: 78). Nevertheless, the government was slow to announce its response to the Nimmo Report. Many of the recommendations were unacceptable to the medical profession. However, government subsidization of those who could not afford to pay medical fees was supported by doctors and, accordingly, a subsidized health-benefits plan was introduced but, despite several adjustments, was not a success. The arrangements were complex, and many people who would have qualified to have their premiums waived or reduced did not seek assistance under the scheme (Kewley 1973: 531–6).

No action was taken on other aspects of the Nimmo Report before the 1969 federal election, at which health insurance was one of the major issues. Labor campaigned strongly on a proposal to introduce a public insurance scheme. The government reaffirmed its commitment to the principles of voluntary insurance but indicated that, if returned to office, it would introduce reforms. The election resulted in a substantial swing against the government and, soon after returning to power, the prime minister called for an urgent review of health policy (Kewley 1973: 509–10).

In 1970, the Minister for Health, Dr A.J. Forbes, announced proposals for reform. Many of the measures were intended to streamline and simplify the insurance system and to increase government control over administration. No changes were made in relation to eligibility for admission to public hospitals. The Nimmo Committee's recommendations for hospitals had such far-reaching implications, the minister said, that the government was not in a position to take action at that time.

The most significant – and the most controversial – proposal related to medical fees. In May 1969, the AMA approved of the concept of the 'most common fee' and, after the 1969 election, published a schedule of fees based on investigations of the fees being charged by doctors. This move was followed by a storm of protest from general practitioners. According to the schedule, specialists were to be paid more than general practitioners for rendering the same services.

The government's objective was to reduce and stabilize the amount paid by patients for each medical service. Under the new arrangements, both Commonwealth and insurance-fund benefits were to be increased so that the out-of-pocket expenses for any service where the most common fee was charged would not exceed $5. Therefore, the success of the plan depended upon a high level of doctor adherence to the schedule of fees. In the face of intense controversy, the prime minister announced that the scheme would go ahead. The government's dilemma is reflected in what Kewley has called the prime minister's 'famous clarification.' In answer to a question about the new plan, Mr Gorton said that

the AMA agrees with us, or I believe will agree with us, that its policy, and it will be its policy to inform patients who ask what the common fee is, and what their own fee is, so that a patient will know whether he is going to be operated on, if that's what it is, on the basis of the common fee or not.' (quoted in Kewley 1973: 509–10)

After some delay the necessary legislation was passed by both Houses of Parliament. The AMA agreed to advise its members to adhere to the fee schedule, which was to be reviewed at two-year intervals. The first review was planned for June 1971. No agreement was reached on a review procedure, but the government hoped that adjustments would be made after negotiations with the profession. In February 1971, however, the AMA unilaterally announced large fee increases. Conflict erupted between the profession and the government, and negotiations failed to reach agreement. The prime minister threatened to introduce a participating-doctor scheme along Canadian lines. This confrontation was cut short by a change of government leadership. The new prime minister, William McMahon, took a more conciliatory attitude towards the AMA. An agreement was reached, and the Minister for Health announced that the new fees would operate for a period of two years. Increasing nonadherence by general practitioners, however, led to a judicial inquiry, after which fees (and the Commonwealth benefit) were increased again in July 1972. The following October, in the midst of preparations for the 1972 election, the government learned that the AMA was planning to announce another round of fee increases to operate from January 1973. The prime minister intervened promptly, and the association agreed not to proceed with its recommendations 'for the time being' (Kewley 1973: 512–25).

Although problems relating to fee-schedule adherence and to the adjustment of fee levels remained unresolved, the introduction of a schedule of fees was of considerable benefit to patients. The majority of doctors adhered to 'the most common fee' and, in conjunction with higher Commonwealth benefits, this fee schedule reduced the out-of-pocket expenses being paid by insured patients, particularly for expensive procedures. However, many of the problems that had been identified by the Nimmo Committee remained. There had been no reform of hospital arrangements. Many low-income earners were still uninsured or held inadequate coverage, and high premium levels continued to cause hardship.[32] Patient co-payments and premiums remained tax deductible. Although the states were running the hospitals and other health services, the formulation of the reform policies had been entirely a Commonwealth matter.

Conclusion

The centralization of power in Australia allowed the Commonwealth to determine the shape of the health-care system in the 1950s and 1960s while taking limited responsibility for health-insurance arrangements. The public subsidization of medical-care costs increased access to medical services, especially for middle-income groups who had not been eligible for membership of friendly societies, but the reintroduction of charges increased barriers to hospital care outside the state of Queensland. The voluntary health-insurance system was designed to achieve the largest possible private sector of medicine with minimum government intervention in the organization and delivery of health services. This reversed the steady trend towards government control of hospital services, which had taken place in all states in the first half of the century. State policy makers were aware that many gaps existed in the services available under a system of predominantly private practice, but the extent to which supplementary services could be provided was limited by financial dependence on the federal government. This situation was exacerbated by Commonwealth policy, which forced the states to meet an increasing share of the operating costs of general hospitals, the most expensive sector of health services. The federal government was able to control by indirect means the provision of medical services in hospitals and the rate at which the states were able to expand other health services.

Commonwealth-government health policy between 1950 and 1972 was both conservative and regressive, a fact which had very little to do with federalism. Non-Labor policy was based on a long-established view of the appropriate role of government in the provision of social services and an equally well-established preference for contributory systems of social insurance. These objectives were compatible with the policy devised by the BMA. The controversy surrounding health policy in the 1960s reflected the polarized nature of the Australian electorate (see table 4 in chapter 8). This division of opinion is manifest in intense competition between the major parties and is one of the major determinants of health policy (Gray 1982: 50).

Non-Labor's long period in office was facilitated by a split in the Labor party in 1955. A Democratic Labor party was formed that was able to direct its perferences to help keep Labor out of office (Emy 1978: 632–3). During this time, the Commonwealth was able to maintain control of a health-insurance system that was of most benefit to its own constituency and to the medical profession. When Labor returned to office in 1972 it inherited an entirely different situation to that of the Labor governments of the 1940s. Policy makers thought that it would be politically impossible to make more than marginal changes in the entrenched system of private, fee-for-service practice. Directly provided services would have to supplement private services rather than replace them. Nevertheless, one element from traditional Labor policy was retained. In the 1970s, the concept of the public hospital, open to all and free for all citizens, was revived.

Australian experience between 1950 and 1970 contrasts with that in Canada in a number of ways. First, the centralization of power in Australia resulted in a situation where major reform could be effected only at the federal level whereas both levels of government contributed to policy development in Canada. Second, where the Commonwealth has the capacity to influence the details of policy, the government of Canada can place only broad conditions on its financial grants to the provinces. Third, the ideological divergence between the major Australian political parties is highlighted by comparison with party politics in Canada. Where the Australian parties promoted policies based on different principles, all parties in Canada came to support the same universal system of health insurance. Although the government of Canada does not have the power to interfere extensively in provincial policy, the underlying consensus of opinion surrounding health policy resulted in much more stable policy development.

Finally, the medical profession in Australia achieved almost all of its objectives between 1950 and 1970 where its Canadian counterpart did not. This situation is a reversal of one of the predictions of 'orthodox' federal theory. In the more decentralized Canadian system, the influence of the medical profession should have been substantial. In Australia, however, the profession not only had access to policy makers, it worked with the government in what Sir Earle Page called a 'cooperative partnership' in the implementation and administration of its own preferred policies. This evidence suggests strongly that the ideologies and orientations of governments and the general pressures within political systems can be far more important than institutional arrangements.

A review of developments in Canada in the post-Medicare period shows that both levels of government continued to contribute to policy. As in the 1940s in Australia, the politics of the period illustrate the difference between formal power and political power. With strong public support, the federal government was able to intervene in health policy despite intense opposition from the provinces.

5

Canadian Health Politics
under National Health Insurance,
1970–86

Health policy in Canada continued to be a highly controversial issue after the introduction of Medicare. Debates entailing a high level of federal-provincial conflict raged about responsibility for financing and about the types of health services that should be promoted. In this process the whole health-care system came under scrutiny. The capacity of both the federal government and provincial governments to find appropriate policy responses was limited by conflicting demands and by the fact that many of these demands had the potential to undermine budgetary objectives. The medical profession opposed increased government intervention, and the public demanded the preservation of universal insurance. There was pressure for a reorganization of the health-care system to de-emphasize curative medical care and to expand the available range of community-based and non-medical services. From the other side of politics, it was suggested that the health-insurance system should be reprivatized.

Despite intergovernmental conflict federalism gave the central government an opportunity to take highly popular policy action to defend universal insurance without incurring the political costs of implementation that fell to the provinces. The policy-making process was federal because Canada's is a federal system. But the policy outcome was the kind of compromise that is familiar in Western democratic systems of government. The demands from the right of politics for reprivatization did not prevail. Nor did governments (outside Quebec) respond to demands from the left for a reorganization of the health-care delivery system. The outcome was what most Canadian governments and most Canadians wanted: health-care expenditures were stabilized, and the universal health-insurance system was preserved and strengthened. However, had the federal government to shoulder all the political responsibility, as in a unitary system, the principles of universality might not have been preserved.

In respect of the capacity of the medical profession to achieve its objectives, the evidence suggests that federalism was a considerable disadvantage. Physicians lost the right to determine their own fees in all Canadian jurisdictions. Government action to control medical fees took place through a series of federal and province-by-province steps that staggered the process over a period of time. A national confrontation with the profession was thus avoided and several provinces were able to take advantage of changed political circumstances that facilitated action. The federal process, rather than enhancing the power of physicians, provided governments with an opportunity to 'divide and rule.'

Health-Care Costs and Proposals for Reform

Total government spending on health services was $0.8 billion in 1949, $1.2 billion in 1955, and $4.4 billion in 1968. As a share of GNP, Canadian health expenditure was 4.35 per cent in 1955, 6.6 per cent in 1968, and 7.49 per cent in 1971 (Hastings 1980: 207; Barer and Evans 1989: 62). By the end of the 1960s, health was a major item in government budgets, and costs were continuing to rise at a faster rate than increases in GNP. Considerable concern developed when a projection of these trends indicated that, 'within the forseeable future, health care would absorb the entire public sector and then the entire economy' (Evans 1982: 330). Such a warning was given by the Economic Council of Canada in 1970, and received wide press coverage (McLeod 1971: 92).

Canadian governments responded by appointing a number of federal and provincial task forces and inquiries that were charged with discovering a means of providing health care at a reasonable and predictable cost. Between 1968 and 1976, ten major inquiries were conducted in Quebec, Nova Scotia, British Columbia, Manitoba, Ontario, and by the federal government. The result was an abundance of information and many proposals for reform of the health-care system.

The first major study was a joint federal-provincial venture set up by the Health Ministers' Conference of 1968. Seven different task forces were established and produced a three-volume set of reports in 1969.[1] The reports generally agreed that there was a need for increased government planning, for the regionalization of responsibility, and for caution in the development of new acute-care facilities (Aucoin 1974: 64–6). A number of recommendations designed to increase the operating efficiency of hospitals were made, including increased use of nurses as substitutes for more highly paid physicians. Emphasis was placed on the need to develop cheaper alternatives to in-hospital care, such as outpatient, domiciliary, day-care, hostel, and transportation services. The recommendations of the report on public health stressed the need for non-institutional services and explored the possibility of establishing community health centres. In contrast with the specific proposals for hospital and public-health services, the reports on medical services were general and recommended only that some experimentation take place in the training of paramedical personnel.

The most important aspect of the task-force reports was that they drew attention to the effects of health insurance. Health insurance, it was realized, promoted the growth of insured services, which were predominantly acute-care hospital services and private medical services.[2] It was argued that this emphasis on insured services led to a lack of experimentation with other forms of delivery in which a wider and less costly range of services might be provided. Insurance also led to the underutilization of health professionals other than physicians (Aucoin 1974: 64–5). The insurance effect is reflected in the percentage of the health budget allocated to the different health sectors. In 1968, 56 per cent of spending was for hospital services; 35 per cent for medical services; 6 per cent for sanitation and waste disposal; and 5 per cent for public health, general standards and controls, research, laboratory services, and personnel training (Hastings 1980: 207). Critics charged that this represented a misallocation of resources that perpetuated an inefficient and unduly expensive system and concentrated on curative rather than preventive health services (McLeod 1971; Weller 1974, 1977). Typical of this view is the following comment:

the existing health delivery system is increasingly recognised as being obsolete and the danger is that health insurance schemes may lock us into paying for an extremely inefficient and costly system ...we have committed ourselves to public payment for health services which are beyond the present public means to control and operated by professional practitioners largely in their own interest ... health remains unorganised, unplanned and fragmented ... its organisational pattern for providing patient care is chaotic at best ... is characterised by persistent shortages of personnel, an oversupply of some types of specialist practitioners and an acute shortage of others ... constant conflict between medical and non-medical practitioners and chronic maldistribution of services. (McLeod 1971: 90–1)

Many of these concerns were repeated and amplified in the other studies of the period. In Manitoba, a White Paper on Health was published in 1972 that recommended the integration of health and social services in regionalized centres and a de-emphasis of acute hospital services. Radical reorganization was proposed in British Columbia through the establishment of a regionalized network of community human-resources and health centres (Foulkes 1973). In Ontario, the report of the Health Planning Task Force (1974) and the health report of the Ontario Economic Council (1976) both stressed that costs, the high use of hospital services, and the maldistribution of health professionals were the main areas needing attention. Recommendations were made for rationalization, regionalization, and the development of non-institutional facilities (Vayda and Deber 1984: 195).

As a result of the recommendations of the federal-provincial task-force reports, two further studies were funded by the federal government. The first concerned the use of nurse practitioners and involved an experimental trial that showed that people accepted this type of service (Hastings and Vayda 1989). The second study investigated the possibility of developing community health centres. It was prompted by mounting evidence from the experience of some prepayment group practices in the United States and from the community health centres in Saskatchewan, which suggested that this form of organization could provide cheaper and more effective health care than could traditional delivery methods (Aucoin 1974: 66–8; Hastings and Vayda 1989).[3] Experience from existing clinics showed a reduced dependence on inpatient hospital services and that a more comprehensive range of preventive and curative services could be provided in 'a broader, people-oriented approach' to health care (Hastings and Vayda 1989).

The report of the Community Health Centre Project to the Health Ministries (1973) recommended that the provinces should establish a wide network of such centres. All health services were to be reorganized and integrated and, through joint federal and provincial action, the system was to be planned, coordinated, and evaluated.

The proposals and ideas in this series of reports, which were prompted by a search for ways to achieve cost-control, shaped the debate on the health-delivery system throughout the 1970s. They were reinforced by a radical critique of therapeutic medicine that emerged in many parts of the world in the 1960s and 1970s and by growing support for a holistic approach to health care. This critique observed that in most Western countries the influence of a medical model of health had grown alongside developments in medical science after the Second World War. Health had come to be seen as a state in which a cure was available for sickness or injury. Public programs were introduced or expanded to increase access to treatment services as a consensus developed that a market allocation of goods that affected matters of life and death was morally unacceptable. According to some interpretations of events, the 1970s mark a turning-point in the priority given to therapeutic medical services. Publications began to appear that urged that the resources being devoted to these services be limited or reduced and that emphasis be placed on policies that would promote health and a healthy environment rather than cure sickness (Illich 1975; Fuchs 1974; McKeown 1976a, 1976b; Starr 1982). Moreover, new ethical problems were raised when it was realized that equal access to the services made possible by modern medical techniques might be beyond the capacities of national economies.[4] For example, it has been estimated that 50,000 Americans would benefit each year from an artificial heart when the technique is perfected. However, the provision of this service would cost between three billion and five billion dollars per year (Bunker 1985: 70).

Canadian policy makers were influenced by these changing ideas and used them to inform and legitimize policy decisions. Research shows that there is little correlation between the amounts spent on personal health services and health outcomes. In 1976, the United States spent 8.6 per cent of GNP on health care, Canada spent 7.2 per cent, and Great Britain spent 5.4 per cent but, as Van Loon (1980: 344) has noted, 'it escaped almost no-one's attention that Great Britain and Canada had very close mortality and morbidity figures, those of the United States were somewhat worse and those of several nations which spent less on health care were considerably better.'

In 1974 the federal government produced an influential report entitled *A New Perspective on the Health of Canadians* (Lalonde 1974). This document attracted considerable attention, both inside and outside Canada.[5] Using the data gathered under universal health insurance, the health status of Canadians was assessed. The conclusion was drawn that increased expenditures on curative health services would yield fewer returns than expenditure in three other areas that influence health: human biology, environment, and life-style. The report proposed a new federal role in these areas, which would be 'a promising new departure' from the previously limited sphere of responsibility.

As a political strategy, the document was cleverly conceived. The new federal role could be both highly visible and inexpensive, and the problem of deciding what to do about the high and increasing cost of curative health services could be left to the provinces. Most important, the report provided a justification for reduced funding for traditional hospital and medical services by both levels of government. As one writer has summarized the legitimation role of the 'New Perspective,' 'if expansion of the health care system could not have much impact on mortality and morbidity, then neither could curtailing its growth. The politically explosive arguments that failure to fund the system at levels professionals declared "needed" would lead to suffering and death could thus be rebuffed. The epidemiologist was recruited to stand beside the accountant in defending the public purse against the clinician' (Evans 1982: 330).

Provincial-Policy Responses to Proposals for the Reorganization of Health Services

The many inquiries and planning reports of the early 1970s furnished governments with information and concrete proposals for action. Changing perceptions of health, statistical information, and the Lalonde Report provided a justification for a reorganization of the health-care delivery system and a shift in funding priorities from hospital and medical services to primary and ambulatory services. Yet, outside Quebec, few of the major recommendations of these reports were implemented. There were, however, piecemeal changes. Some of the proposals of the Foulkes Report were implemented by an NDP government in British Columbia between 1973 and 1975 but they were not in operation long enough to become established, and most were dismantled after a Social Credit government was returned to power in 1975 (Clague et al 1984).[6] Health and social services were integrated in Manitoba, and to a lesser extent in Nova Scotia, in the 1970s (Hastings and Vayda 1989). By 1983, twenty-eight health centres of various kinds had been established in Ontario, and there were nineteen in other provinces outside Quebec. Home-care services were expanded rapidly but not in the planned way recommended by many of the reports (Hastings and Vayda 1989). Regionalization and decentralization of responsibility for some services were introduced in all provinces, but only Quebec transferred a degree of financial control to regional bodies. Community participation in decision making increased slowly, and, in several provinces, there is lay representation on the governing bodies of the major health professions (Hastings and Vayda 1989). Overall, however, little was done to change the organization of the health system other than in the province of Quebec, and innovative policy making along the lines suggested in most of the reports has not taken place.

In Quebec, however, a radical reorganization of the health system was undertaken. These developments are examined in chapter 7.

Provincial reluctance to take an active role in the planning and organization of the health system is not a by-product of institutional arrangements, however. There are no constitutional obstacles to provincial action, and, in health, the provinces are regarded as the senior level of government. The reasons are to be found in a range of constraints that would be present whatever the system of government.

The first and most important constraint was the opposition of the medical profession to almost all of the proposals. Physicians vehemently opposed any alteration of the fee-for-service system of remuneration. Group-practice prepayment plans and community health centres in the United States and Saskatchewan are staffed by salaried doctors, a system that was suggested for the proposed centres. The profession opposed regionalization, which might allow a planned distribution of services and might give governments more control over hospital expenditures. In a regionalized system a fixed budget may be allocated to local hospital boards, which are then responsible for deficits and for any reduction in facilities, creating a buffer between the hospital system and government. Lay representation on the profession's governing boards was resisted but not with the same intensity as were other proposals. The increased use of paramedical and other health and social-welfare professionals has the potential to undermine the bargaining position of the profession and might intensify the emergent challenge to medical dominance. The profession's resistance to any suggestion that the numbers of doctors being trained should be reduced is a response to this threat, and the rapid increase in the doctor/population ratio in the 1970s reduced the likelihood that other health professionals would be engaged as substitutes for doctors. Second, provincial hospital associations did not welcome a transfer of resources to non-institutional settings, and hospitals opposed the establishment of regional and community boards as planning agencies (Hastings and Vayda 1989). Third, many of these proposals offered only the prospect of long-term gains for governments. The substitution of expensive services and facilities with less expensive forms would be a slow process and would require attitudinal as well as organizational changes. Compared with the introduction of health insurance, for example, benefits to the electorate are not highly visible and are difficult to explain. Such benefits as did accrue might be offset by administrative difficulties and by inconvenience for users of established services. Moreover, there was concern that the establishment of new services would merely become an addition to existing services, thus increasing rather than reducing costs (Weller 1974: 110–11; Hastings and Vayda 1989). Finally, there was no widespread public demand for community-based services, which were largely unknown and untried: the proposals were made by experts and professionals. Thus the major obstacles to policy innovation were the familiar problems of political opposition, budgetary concerns, and lack of support for new policies. Institutional arrangements were not a major constraint.

During this period, it was suggested that intergovernmental financial arrangements be changed. It was argued that the cost-shared method of funding provided little incentive for provincial governments to develop alternative services. Under cost-sharing approximately half of the costs of existing services were met by the federal government, whereas the full cost of new uninsured services had to be met by the provinces. The change to block funding in 1977 was not followed by any significant departure from existing policies, however, and provincial governments continued to pursue courses that would achieve short-term budgetary aims[7] within the limits of the political constraints. All provinces had the same opportunities as Quebec to intervene in the organization of the health system. The important difference was that Quebeckers elected a series of activist nationalist governments committed to social-policy reform where other Canadians did not.

The Response of the Federal Government to Rising Health Costs

In 1970, the federal government devised a means of controlling the rate of growth of its own share of health-care funding. Cost-sharing, over which it had little control, was to be replaced by block funding under which a fixed per-capita grant based on current expenditures would be adjusted annually according to the rate of growth of GNP. It was five years before agreement was reached with the provinces on the federal proposal because health-care costs stabilized between 1971 and 1975. During this time, no serious attempt was made to alter existing arrangements, but, when costs again rose rapidly in 1975, new agreements were negotiated very quickly.

In a federal system, the need to arrive at acceptable arrangements for the sharing of finances adds an extra dimension to the policy-making process, if only to the extent that it provides an arena in which regional governments can voice their claims. While governments may refuse to compromise and so obstruct action, in practice instances of this are rare.

In the 1976 negotiations a compromise was reached between the large provinces and the federal government. The poorer provinces were not able to obstruct the change to block funding but they were compensated with a greater degree of equalization than had previously been in place. The evidence suggests that financial negotiations in a federal system are a more public version of the bargaining over resources that takes place in all political systems. During the negotiations, concerns about health policy were entirely subordinated to financial considerations. This reflected the preoccupation with budgetary problems at a time of slow economic growth, a feature shared by unitary and non-unitary systems of government in the 1970s and 1980s.

The Established Programs Financing Act, 1977[8]

The introduction of Established-Programs Financing (EPF) in 1977 was part of a long adjustment process to rationalize federal-provincial financial relations that had been in train since the 1950s. Largely in response to the demands of the province of Quebec for more control over policies within provincial jurisdiction, the Established Programs (Interim Arrangements) Act was passed by the federal government in 1965. Under this act, any province could elect to 'opt out' of cost-sharing agreements for established programs and receive instead a transfer of tax points on the condition that the program continue unchanged. Only Quebec accepted the offer, opting out of hospital cost-sharing arrangements and four other social-policy programs (Brown 1984: 17–18). Other provinces feared that acceptance of the offer might lead to lower levels of federal funding (Brown 1983: 49).

This change had two main consequences. It established the idea that, once a program was operating successfully, a more limited federal policy role might be appropriate. Second, it set a precedent: the richer provinces could argue more strongly that raising their own taxes was a constitutional right[9] and that opting-out arrangements were a feasible alternative to the conditional grant.

The first definite proposals concerning a change from cost-sharing to block funding were put to the provinces in 1971. Other than retention of the five 'national standards' there would be no conditions. Ontario, Quebec, and Alberta proposed that the federal government transfer tax points rather than pay the grant in cash. No agreement was reached, and during the next four years the proposals 'remained under consideration without much sense of urgency' (Van Loon 1980: 344).

A sharp increase in costs in 1975, however, led to very quick action. The proposals of 1971 were revived, hasty negotiations took place, and new arrangements were entered into in 1976. The compromise reached between Alberta, Ontario, Quebec, and the federal government was that half of the grant should be paid in cash and that the other half should take the form of transferred tax points. An additional grant of $20 per capita, to be adjusted annually by the same formula as the block grant, was made to the provinces to promote the expansion of non-institutional services.

The provinces were aware that the federal government had the power to place a ceiling on increases in its share of funding, whether agreement was reached or not. Serious matters, such as expenditure control and the sharing of tax points, usually take precedence over the political grandstanding frequently involved in the politics of federalism. As one writer has described the regular five-year review of Canadian financial arrangements,

the negotiations leading up to the revisions ... resemble an elaborate pantomime with the federal government represented by the Minister of Finance and the provincial governments represented by treasurers attacking them from various angles until all dissolves in apparent disarray only a few months before the critical deadline. In this Canadian version of the Perils of Pauline, the stage is set for the prime minister and premiers to meet at the last minute and after a certain amount of posturing, snatch forth an agreement, saving Canada from yet another crisis. (Van Loon 1980: 351–2)

This account may underplay the intensity of the conflict that sometimes exists between the federal government and some provinces but unless, as in 1945–6, a particularly hard-line position is adopted by one or more parties there is considerable room for compromise. In the case of the EPF negotiations, despite a variety of different concerns and positions among the provinces, acceptable arrangements were negotiated.[10] The compromise on the combination of cash payments and ceded tax points reached between the larger provinces and the federal government has been mentioned. The position of Manitoba was unclear, but the other six provinces were opposed to block funding.[11] British Columbia objected to the proposed ceiling on funding increases (Brown 1984: 27–8). Saskatchewan was opposed because the government thought that a reduced federal role might lead to an erosion of the 'national standards' (Weller and Manga 1983: 23). The Atlantic provinces, with their small revenue bases, regarded tax points as a poor substitute for cost-sharing arrangements. Heavily dependent on transfers and on equalization payments, these provinces opposed any decrease in federal financial power, while the richer provinces tried to limit the amount of money 'drained to the poorer provinces through what they view as a federal siphon' (Van Loon 1980: 351). The new arrangements provided for greater equalization between the provinces. Under cost-sharing, provinces that spent less on hospital services received lower per-capita federal contributions. Under EPF, payments to the poorer provinces were increased and payments to the richer provinces were decreased so that, after a three-year phasing-in period, per-capita payments to all provinces were equal (Taylor 1989: 16). Money, of course, is infinitely divisible, and the result was a set of agreements that all parties could accept.

Provincial Policy Making and the Control of Health-Care Expenditures

With the change to block funding, the provinces were faced with the task of keeping increases in health-care costs in line with the rate of growth of GNP or of meeting additional expenditures without assistance from the federal government. However, an unintended consequence of EPF was to increase the amount of federal funding for health care, but this did not alter the provinces' record in meeting cost-containment objectives. Although there was some variation from year to year, both before and after the change to EPF, Canadian health expenditures were stabilized throughout the 1970s.

One of the cost-control mechanisms employed related to the rate of increase in medical fee schedules in the 1970s. After a period of 'extraordinary income gains' in the late 1960s, increases in provincial fee schedules were held below the rate of inflation between 1971 and 1976, falling in real terms by 20 per cent. In the late 1970s increases were held in line with inflation but the rate rose in the early 1980s (Barer and Evans 1989: 77–84). Thus provincial governments, unlike Australian federal governments, were able to exert a considerable degree of control over increases in doctor's fees.

Although there was no deliberate attempt outside Quebec to restructure medical-practice patterns, cost-containment policies aimed at reducing the use of acute hospital facilities indirectly had this effect. Through a mechanism known as 'global budgeting,' hospital boards were given a fixed budget from which to meet expenditures.[12] In response to this financial pressure, the number of acute-care hospital beds was reduced. In 1970, there were 5.6 short-term beds per thousand of population. In 1975, this ratio had been reduced to 5.2, and in 1978–9 further reduced to 4.8.[13] This policy continued into the 1980s (Barer and Evans 1989: 98–108).

At the same time that hospital facilities were being reduced, the number of physicians in Canada was rapidly increasing. Whereas in 1970 there was one doctor for every 689 people, by 1983 the ratio had increased to 1 for 512 (Van Loon 1980: 347; Barer and Evans 1989: 86). The result is that there has been a decline in the number of beds available to each physician. Services to inpatients have become a decreasing share of medical practice whereas primary-care services make up a larger share (Barer and Evans 1989: 147–8). Thus, some movement away from expensive high-technology, curative medical services has been achieved as a by-product of cost-control measures. Such changes have the potential to alter significantly patterns of medical practice if sustained in the long term.

By 1979, financial restrictions led to pressures that made health policy again a highly controversial issue. The medical profession charged that both levels of government were 'underfunding' the system. The provinces accused the federal government of reduced financial support, and the federal government said the provinces were diverting federal funds away from the system. Consumer, welfare, and women's groups, trade unions, and the Canadian Nurses Association mobilized in defence of 'universal Medicare.' After five years of controversy, the Canada Health Act was passed in 1984. The act empowers the federal government to withhold federal funds from provinces in which the five national standards are not upheld.

During the period leading up to the passage of the Canada Health Act, federal-provincial relations were very strained. The division of responsibility for health-care financing allowed the two levels of government to blame each other for the perceived shortcomings of the system. The federal government was held responsible by consumer groups for not enforcing the national standards while the provinces were held responsible for permitting extra-billing and, in some cases, for introducing user charges. Notwithstanding their different responsibilities, the constraints operating on both levels of government were similar. Both wanted to maintain pressure on increasing health costs, both were opposed by the medical profession, and both were held responsible by citizens for aspects of policy. There was no easy solution to this policy predicament.

The Politics of Cost Containment

The response to pressure on medical incomes by government cost-containment policies was an increase in the number of doctors who 'opted out' of the insurance plans and/or 'extra-billed' their patients.[14] The extent of this practice varied considerably from province to province. There was no extra-billing in British Columbia or Quebec and very little in New Brunswick, Newfoundland, and Prince Edward Island. In 1980, the number of doctors charging more than the schedule fee was 12 per cent in Nova Scotia, 5 per cent in Saskatchewan, 16 per cent in Ontario, and 23 per cent in Alberta (*Montreal Gazette* 4 September 1980). While these percentages are not large, extra-billing doctors were not randomly distributed but were concentrated geographically and by specialty, with the result that it was difficult in some areas to find an 'opted-in' specialist to which low-income patients could be referred (Naylor 1982: 13). For example, in 1982, 62 per cent of Ontario's anaesthetists, 43 per cent of opthalmologists, and 39 per cent of gynaecologists were 'opted-out' (Grossman 1982).

In order to help meet their budgetary targets or for ideological reasons, a few provinces began to impose or to threaten to impose direct charges for hospital services. When national hospital insurance was introduced, Alberta and British Columbia were making small direct charges to patients. This practice continued under cost-sharing but the amounts raised were deducted from the federal contribution. The move to block funding allowed the provinces to increase revenue from hospital fees without a reduction in federal funds. Charges were introduced or increased in British Columbia, Alberta, and Newfoundland. There were no charges in Saskatchewan, Nova Scotia, New Brunswick, or Prince Edward Island, and the three other provinces charged only for long-term patients. User charges became controversial largely because Alberta, for ideological reasons, announced its intention to introduce a substantial hospital fee in 1983.

The Canada Health Act 1984

The erosion of the principles of Medicare first became a major political issue in the 1979 election campaign. Both NDP leader Ed Broadbent and Prime Minister Trudeau accused the provinces of diverting federal health funds to other sectors. Mr Broadbent called for a return to cost-sharing, under which, he said, the provinces would again be forced to spend a dollar for every dollar contributed by Ottawa.[15] Mr Trudeau said that this policy would be considered if the provinces persisted in allowing extra-billing. The Progressive Conservative party governments of Ontario,

Manitoba, Alberta, and New Brunswick were singled out for criticism, creating difficulties for federal Conservative leader Joe Clark, who sought to avoid the issue (*Globe and Mail* 25 April 1979: 1). In response to NDP pressure in the House of Commons, finance minister Jean Chrétien said that it was a provincial responsibility to provide enough money to keep doctors in Medicare. Health minister Monique Bégin said a federal-provincial conference might be the best way of clarifying the Medicare guidelines but warned that federal payments could be withdrawn if 'the spirit of Medicare' were not upheld (*Globe and Mail* 20 March 1979: 1). The reaction of the provinces was relatively mild at this time, but only the NDP government of Saskatchewan supported the federal position.[16]

The federal government was defeated in June 1979, and the Progressive Conservative party came to power. Although the party had made no firm statement on Medicare during the campaign, the new Health minister, David Crombie, said that his party had a clear 'commitment to Medicare, not only in terms of financial obligations, but in terms of philosophy' (*Toronto Star* 5 June 1979: 1). He called a federal-provincial Health ministers' conference for the following September at which he told his provincial counterparts that he wanted to work towards national standards for Medicare. The conference decided that a review of the health system should be undertaken. It was agreed to appoint Mr Justice Hall, former Supreme Court judge and chairman of the Royal Commission on Health Services (1961–4), to conduct an inquiry (*Globe and Mail* 18 September 1979: 1).

In the meantime, citizen groups had mobilized to 'defend universal Medicare.' Health Coalition groups were organized, and a number of provincial conferences were held. In Alberta, an organization known as 'Friends of Medicare' was formed. In November 1979, a national conference, which the organizers called 's.o.s. Medicare,' was held. A federal organization, the Canadian Health Coalition, was set up. This body receives financial support from member organizations and from the Canadian Labour Council, and has its headquarters at the Canadian Labour Congress building in Ottawa. It represents a variety of welfare, consumer, church, trade-union, and women's groups, including hospital-employee associations and the Canadian Council of Social Development.[17] The organization is 'dedicated to saving Medicare and to improving the health care system' and, in 1985, represented over 2.5 million Canadians. Throughout the early 1980s, the activities of the coalition and its member bodies, supported by national and provincial NDP parties and provincial Liberal parties, kept opposition to reprivatization on the political agenda. Dur-

.... iis campaign, 'the-most-talked-about Medicare system in the country' was the Quebec system, which reformers wanted implemented in the rest of Canada. The demands were 'no extra-billing, no premiums, no user-fees' (CMA *Journal* 130 [1984]: 63). In 1985, the coalition was still active, conducting a 'Monitor Medicare' campaign, which involved a wide range of political and information-dissemination activities (Canadian Health Coalition 1985).

The minority Conservative government did not survive and, in February 1980, the Liberal party was returned to office. Madame Bégin again became Minister for National Health and Welfare, a portfolio that she describes as 'the worst of all possible worlds in the early 1980s.' She decided to wait for the report of the Hall inquiry before taking action, but her aim was to achieve a health system in which there would be 'no charge at the point of service.'[18] Although the Canada Health Act was clearly motivated by political concerns, officials at the Department of National Health and Welfare and members of the NDP confirm that the minister was strongly committed to the preservation of Medicare.[19]

The report of Special Commissioner Hall was presented in September 1980 and met with wide approval, except from the medical profession and provincial Health ministers. He reported that 'I found no one, not any Government or individual not the Medical Profession nor any organisation, not in favour of Medicare. There were differences of opinion, it is true, on how it should be organized and provided but no one wanted it terminated' (Hall 1980: 2). He found evidence 'from one end of Canada to the other that extra-billing by physicians ... was unacceptable. The opposition to these practices came from Government as well as from individuals and consumer groups however ... virtually all ... were equally forthright in advocating that physicians were entitled to be adequately compensated' (Hall 1980: 25). The commissioner argued that neither governments nor the medical profession should have the right to unilaterally determine fees and that disputes should be referred to binding arbitration. He recommended that extra-billing be eliminated. Studies done for the commission showed that it inhibited 'reasonable' access to services (Hall 1980: 27-9).

The commissioner was critical of the 'user-pay' concept and of the closure of certain kinds of hospital wards. The suggestion in a number of briefs that there be a return to a free-market health system was rejected on grounds of administrative costs alone. U.S. experience was drawn upon to demonstrate the additional administrative costs that could be expected to follow reprivatization (Hall 1980: 42-3).

On the question of funding, it was found that, under EPF, the federal contribution had not fallen but, in fact, had risen from 39.7 per cent of all health expenditures in 1975–6 to 44.7 per cent in 1979–80. Nor was the allegation that 'federal health dollars were being diverted' established. The commissioner argued that one of the purposes of the change to EPF was that the provinces should have more autonomy in health-resource allocation. He took the view that only the cash portion of the federal contribution was a conditional grant. The cash grant was being allocated to the health sector (Hall 1980: 11–17).[20]

Controversy had also arisen over the question of insurance premiums, which were still collected in British Columbia, Alberta, and Ontario. All other provinces had moved to tax-based methods of financing. The question was whether failure to pay premiums should deprive residents of coverage and was compounded by the fact that, as in Australia in the early 1970s, many low-income earners did not know of their right to be exempted from the obligation to pay. The commissioner recommended that the three provinces concerned should gradually move away from the premium system (Hall 1980: 41, 44–6).

Despite the wide support for federal action based on the recommendations of the Hall Commission, major constraints remained. Federal-provincial relations had been strained for some time. There had been conflict over constitutional reform throughout the 1970s, and controversy over energy policy. Antagonistic federal-provincial relations were widely thought to be a political liability for the federal government, and many politicians sought to avoid further confrontation.[21]

In the atmosphere of recession, there was growing support for neo-conservative ideas, and suggestions that the health system be partly or fully reprivatized were increasingly made. A report to the Ontario government in 1978, prepared by public servants and members of the medical profession, recommended 'deterrent fees' for hospital patients, increased premiums, and extra-billing. It was argued that consumers would thereby be made more aware of the cost of services (*Winnipeg Free Press* 14 January 1978: 8). A professor of medicine from the University of Toronto wrote a complete condemnation of public health insurance and, in 1978, in company with Dr Peter Arnold, president of the General Practitioner's Society of Australia, he conducted a lecture tour of the United States (*Globe and Mail* 26 November 1978: 10). The Fraser Institute, an independent research organization in Vancouver, produced a similar critique in 1979, calling for government withdrawal and a return to private insurance and market forces.

In addition to provincial opposition and the influence of neo-conservative ideas, there were legal and constitutional problems in the way of federal action. The five national standards had not been clearly defined in previous legislation with the result that there was difficulty in determining what constituted a breach of the conditions. Moreover, there was doubt about whether the attachment of conditions to the block grant was constitutionally valid. There were limits, too, on the ways in which the federal government could intervene. Under cost-sharing, it had been possible to withhold a portion of the federal funds, whereas, under EPF, a federal penalty had to take the form of withholding the whole grant. The only other alternative was the passage of new legislation. Officials of the Department of Health and Welfare were unable to devise less visible proposals.[22]

On the release of the Hall Report, the federal minister called a Health ministers' conference. The provinces dismissed the Hall recommendations out of hand.[23] The general view was that the abolition of extra-billing would create more problems than it would solve. The three provinces collecting premiums were strongly opposed to the suggestion that other forms of revenue collection be substituted (*Montreal Gazette* 1 September 1980: 10).

One of the most powerful opponents of federal intervention was the Health minister of Alberta, David Russell, whose influence was enhanced by his position as chairman of the provincial Health ministers' conferences in the early 1980s. His opposition and that of the British Columbian Health minister were largely ideological. Mr Russell's support for reprivatization did not arise from budgetary difficulties. High oil and gas revenues had led to a situation in which it appeared that, after federal transfers, Alberta had a greater fiscal capacity than the federal government in the late 1970s (Brown 1984: 72–3). In response to the Hall Report, Mr Russell said that Medicare premiums were an important philosophical element in Alberta's health system and that, while the province could certainly afford to abolish them, it had no intention of doing so (*Globe and Mail* 5 September 1980: 1). Two months earlier, premiums had been raised by 15 per cent, and the minister further announced that he intended to introduce legislation giving doctors the right to opt out of the provincial insurance plan (*Globe and Mail* 5 September 1980: 1). Few of Mr Russell's proposals were implemented but they gained wide publicity and added legitimacy to the arguments of other proponents of reprivatization.

Throughout 1981, the Medicare issue continued to simmer. The three provinces concerned raised their premium levels. The CMA and its provincial divisions marked the anniversary of the Hall Report by holding 'strategy sessions' but no details of plans for action were made public (*Globe and Mail* 3 September 1981: 8). At its 1981 annual general meeting, the CMA resolved to step up the pressure being placed on parliamentarians to promote the 'demonopolization' of Medicare by government and to study and develop possible means of obtaining additional finance from the private sector. The theme was that 'doctors are not extra-billing – governments are under-funding' (*Globe and Mail* 25 August 1981: L1).

Early in 1981, the federal government appointed an all-party parliamentary task force to enquire into federal-provincial financial arrangements. The history of fiscal federalism, EPF and its consequences, the health system, and the other jointly funded social programs were examined. Like Commissioner Hall, the task force held public hearings in all provinces, received a large number of written briefs, and consulted with all provincial governments.

The task force report, *Fiscal Federalism in Canada* (Breau Report 1981), recognized the inextricable relationship between all the contested health-policy issues. It reported that 'the question of "underfunding" is linked to the supply of physicians and physician's incomes, that in turn, to the problem of extra-billing (and the question of the inefficient utilization of health resources) and that again to concerns for erosion of program conditions, particularly those of accessibility and universality' (Breau Report 1981: 97). On the question of health-care funding, the task force recommended that existing arrangements be continued on the grounds that federal funding reductions would lead to increased privatization and ultimately to higher costs (Breau Report 1981: 114–15).

The appropriate policy-role of the federal government, it was decided, should be to formulate, monitor, and enforce the five conditions without becoming directly involved in provincial policy. Hospital user charges were rejected for reasons of both principle and practicality. Studies showed that 'user-charges that are high enough to serve as deterrent fees deter the wrong people (the old and the poor for the most part) while user-charges which are low enough to be acceptable on distributional grounds, are too low to be worth collecting – administrative costs more than match any revenue gains' (Breau Report 1981: 108).

The only issue on which the three-party committee divided was extra-billing. The two Conservative party members did not agree with the four Liberals and the one New Democrat that the practice should be banned. They were prepared only to recommend that, if physicians wished to opt out, they must do so for all patients. This proposal would have had the effect of reducing extra-billing because opted-out doctors would be able to treat only patients who were prepared to pay an extra charge.

All members of the task force agreed that action should be taken to clarify and enforce the five conditions. It was recommended that intergovernmental negotiations be initiated but that, if such negotiations failed to reach agreement, federal funds should be withheld from the provinces that did not meet the conditions as interpreted by the task force (Breau Report 1981: 115–16).

In the tense atmosphere that prevailed at the time, it seemed highly unlikely that negotiations would be successful. Nevertheless, a federal position paper was prepared and a federal-provincial Health ministers' conference was called. In the meantime, physician militancy increased in several provinces, and a series of work stoppages took place in Ontario. The *Globe and Mail* (30 April 1982: 3) reported that Mme Bégin was 'keeping a safe distance' from the disputes in a deliberate effort not to provoke further hostilities. The minister spoke 'in conciliatory tones' of the forthcoming conference, it was reported, and said that she 'hoped some consensus would develop without her prompting' (*Globe and Mail* 30 April 1982: 3). A month before the conference, the minister lost her one provincial ally when the NDP government of Saskatchewan was defeated.

The May meeting totally broke down. The federal position paper was presented at 'a polite but cool morning session.' Heated and angry debates took place over lunch and the meeting ended after one day instead of the scheduled two (*Globe and Mail* 27 May 1982: 1). Despite this débâcle, the federal position paper was redrafted and presented to another Health ministers' conference in the following September. No progress was made, however, and the provinces issued a press statement threatening a constitutional challenge if the federal government attempted to pass new legislation.

The controversy escalated during the remainder of 1982 and throughout 1983. Massive publicity and lobbying campaigns were launched by all medical associations. The president of the CMA, Dr Marc Baltzan, and Mme Bégin became prominent media figures. The lines of battle were the provincial Health ministers and the medical associations, on the one hand, against the federal government, provincial Liberal parties, all NDP parties, women's groups, trade unions, consumer associations, and the national and provincial health coalitions, on the other (Taylor 1989: 30–1). To the federal minister the problem seemed to have no solution. Her attempts to gain agreement on voluntary control of extra charges had failed. She felt that no one took her position seriously, and doubts about the degree of Cabinet support she enjoyed were expressed publicly. In the minister's opinion the Liberal party was 'fragmented and dying.' It had 'no platform, no ideas and no policies.' There were rumours that the prime minister was about to resign, and preliminary leadership struggles were underway. Many members of Cabinet and the party appeared to Mme Bégin to be influenced by neo-conservative ideas and were not opposed to the introduction of user-charges. Until 1983, the minister was uncertain of the prime minister's position on the issue.[24]

The turning-point came in March 1983. Premiums were raised by 47 per cent in Alberta, and Health minister David Russell announced that a hospital fee of $20 per day would be introduced, which would 'give Alberta the first universal system of hospital fees in the country.' He issued a direct challenge to the federal government, saying that, if the federal minister retaliated, 'Alberta would fight back' (*Globe and Mail* 29 March 1983: 11). A study of the Alberta health system showed that, although the negotiated schedule fee had increased by 50 per cent in three years, extra-billing had also increased rapidly. It was further shown that doctors 'were extra-billing thousands of senior citizens, welfare recipients and low income earners' (Taylor 1989: 31).

Senior officials at the Department of National Health and Welfare identify the Alberta announcement as the stimulus for determined federal action. The minister privately consulted three top constitutionalists. Their opinion was that the federal government had the power to enforce compliance with the five conditions. The Department of Justice was then asked to give an official opinion. This, too, was positive, and was made public in May 1983. Proposals for new legislation were then taken to the Policy and Planning Committee of Cabinet, which was chaired by the prime minister. No decision was made. The Minister of Health remained uncertain about the support of several key ministers, and she attributes reluctance to take action to concern about the prestige and 'political clout' of the medical profession. In fact, only a month before the federal decision to proceed with legislation was announced publicly, the prime minister is reported to have said in a newspaper interview that 'economic sanctions against delinquent provinces were unreasonable' (*CMA Journal* 130 [1 January 1984]: 61).

The next step in the minister's strategy was to commission a number of opinion polls in six provinces. She told the press that the surveys showed that there was 'overwhelming support for banning health care user-fees' (*Toronto Star* 23 June 1983: A10). Details of the findings do not appear to have been made public at the time. However, in September

1983, a national poll showed that 85 per cent of Canadians supported Medicare, rating it one of the most important government services; 56 per cent of people were opposed to extra-billing; 17 per cent thought doctors were justified in charging extra in some cases; and 16 per cent supported extra-billing. The findings on hospital user charges were similar: 54 per cent opposed, 13 per cent in favour, and 17 per cent of the opinion that charges might be justified in limited cases (*Calgary Herald* 12 September 1983: A1).[25] In August, Mr Russell announced that the introduction of the proposed Alberta hospital charges would be delayed. Two days earlier, a Gallup poll had shown that Canadians, including Albertans, favoured an increase in taxes rather than the imposition of fees to cover health-care costs (*Calgary Herald* 26 August 1983: A5).

Mme Bégin attributes a sudden change in Cabinet to the opinion poll findings. Many members now urged that action be taken quickly.[26] The issue was seen as one which might help to improve the very low electoral standing of the government while placing the Conservative opposition in a difficult situation. During the following six months, the policy of the opposition was unclear and its statements were evasive.

A white paper, entitled *Preserving Universal Medicare*, was released in July 1983. It concentrated on the question of direct charges to patients and announced that a new Canada Health Act would be introduced into Parliament in the fall. The legislation was portrayed as 'the next step in a quarter century of effort to guarantee that every resident of Canada has access to insured services on a fully pre-paid basis ... the erosion of Medicare is sufficiently widespread to constitute a national problem ... We cannot preserve Medicare by charging the sick ... We can only preserve Medicare by ensuring its basic principles' (Government of Canada 1983: 33).

Reactions to the paper followed established divisions on the issue. Neither the leaders of the federal opposition nor the health critic (shadow minister) were available for comment. Social-development critic, Flora MacDonald, said that the party favoured 'some sort of disincentive' but would not expand on Conservative party policy. A spokesperson for the Ontario Medical Association said that the minister was 'just making another grandstand play' (*Toronto Star* 26 July 1983: A9).

Those who hoped that the federal government would not proceed were to be disappointed. The following September, the minister met with her provincial counterparts. She told them that the new Canada Health Act was about to receive Cabinet approval, after which the provinces would be supplied with a copy of the legislation. The purpose of the act was to eliminate extra charges, and the only point that was negotiable was the time that would be allowed to reach the goal (*Toronto Star* 8 September 1984: A3).

Soon after the legislation was introduced into Parliament, the federal Conservative party announced that it supported the act. The Treasurer of Ontario said that he wished that the federal party had supported the provincial position, but there was otherwise little public comment from provincial governments (*Toronto Star* 15 December 1983: 1). The response of the medical profession was to adopt a much more conciliatory attitude. Two days after the Conservative party decision, the CMA announced that it wanted to take 'a non-confrontational approach and a negotiations approach to the Canada Health Act' and would like to 'talk things over' with the Health minister (*Toronto Star* 17 December 1983: 1). With all-party support for the legislation before the House of Commons, those wishing to influence the passage of the act had limited opportunities to do so.

The Canada Health Act passed the second reading stage in January 1984. Extensive public hearings were held in the committee stage. Minor amendments were made at the request of the NDP, but the party failed to achieve its two major aims, which were to have the definition of insured services broadened to include non-physician services and to have the financial penalties for non-compliance with the act substantially increased. At the request of the CMA, the Conservative party moved an amendment that provided for binding arbitration in the event of disputes over fee schedules. The CMA saw this 'as some compensation for the probable loss of the right to extra-bill' (*CMA Journal* 132 [15 January 1985]: 171–2). A storm of protest issued from provincial governments, which wanted to retain full control over the process by which schedule fee levels were negotiated. The Ontario Health minister said that federal politicians of all parties were 'euchred' by the CMA, and the British Columbia Health minister said the change in the act was 'one of the few great accomplishments of 1984. They were able to amend it and make it worse' (*Globe and Mail* 5 April 1984: 5).

The Canada Health Act was passed unanimously in the House of Commons on 9 April 1984, and in the Senate on 17 April, after provincial Health ministers had made an unprecedented appearance in the Senate in a final attempt to block the legislation (*Globe and Mail* 5 April 1986: 5). The provisions of the act became effective on 1 July. In the same month, Mme Bégin announced her retirement from politics.

At the federal election in September 1984, the Liberal party suffered its worst defeat in Canadian history, and the Conservative party took office with a very large majority. Federal-government policy, however, did not change. The new minister, Jake Epp, announced that Medicare 'was a sacred trust' and would be preserved (*Toronto Star* 7 September 1984: A15). The Mulroney government continued to apply the provisions of the Canada Health Act. One by one, the provinces took action to eliminate extra-billing. By September 1985, all doctors were within the insurance system in Nova Scotia, Prince Edward Island, Manitoba, and Saskatchewan. Negotiations were sometimes tense but there were no strikes. In Alberta, Mr Russell announced that, although he had no intention of banning extra-billing, the numbers of doctors charging more than the schedule fee had dropped from 43.4 per cent in 1982 to 25 per cent in 1985[27] (*Calgary Herald* 4 June 1985: B12).

The Conservative party of Ontario lost government in June 1985 for the first time in forty-two years. The Liberal party formed a minority government. After considerable debate within the NDP, it was decided not to enter into coalition with the Liberals. Agreement was reached between the parties on a two-year 'accord.' Committed to preserving Medicare and in need of NDP support, the government introduced legislation to ban extra-billing in December 1985 amid a storm of protest from the Ontario Medical Association (OMA), which represents most of the province's doctors. The government had previously attempted to negotiate with the OMA and was ready to offer certain benefits, such as higher fees and improved conditions of sabbatical leave, in return for agreement to eliminate extra-billing. The OMA, however, refused to participate in discussions.[28] Unable to negotiate a settlement, the government proceeded with legislation that provided for fines of up to $10,000 in the event of default. The passage of the legislation was stormy. Public hearings were held in the committee stage and attracted wide publicity. Negotiations between the government and the OMA finally commenced in March. A variety of compensatory offers were made to the profession, including control of the $100 million that Ottawa would return if extra-billing were eliminated (*Globe and Mail* 11 April 1986: A5; 16 April 1986: A9; 22 April 1986: A6; 14 May 1986: 1; 26 May 1986: A8; 30 May 1986). The May budget contained a new allocation of $850 million for hospital construction, a reversal of the cost-containment policies of the previous decade. The two sides, however, failed to reach agreement, and the OMA voted to hold a province-wide strike, which began on 11 June. The government did not withdraw the legislation as requested by the profession, and Bill 94 became law on 20 June 1986.

Between August 1985 and June 1986 public support for legislation to prohibit extra-billing fell from 72 per cent to 54 per cent, a reflection of the success of the doctor's campaign (*Globe and Mail* 2 July 1986: A2). The political difficulties of the government were serious: during the dispute only 37 per cent of people approved of the way the government was handling the situation. However, 77 per cent of people disapproved of the strike, and 54 per cent thought that the government should order the doctors to return to work (*Globe and Mail* 27 June 1984: 1). After two weeks, a polarization of opinion developed within the profession and in early July, it became clear that physician support for the strike was declining. OMA-organized marches and meetings drew smaller-than-expected numbers, and doctors in some areas began to reopen their offices and to return to their hospital posts (*Globe and Mail* 27 June 1986: A1, A27; 3 July 1986: 1, A17). On 4 July, after a day-long meeting at which one member said there had been 250 generals, 'each of whom was sure his plan was the best,' the OMA voted to call off the strike. The president said the association had been 'getting nowhere against a provincial government that would not budge' and had failed to get its message across to the public. He said, however, that the OMA would continue to fight and refused to rule out another strike (*Globe and Mail* 5 July 1986: 1, A2, A16). Ten days later, federal Health minister Jake Epp announced that $115 million in withheld funds would be returned to the Ontario government (*Globe and Mail* 14 July 1986: 1, A2).

In the meantime, several important changes had taken place in Alberta. Mr Russell moved from the Health portfolio, the province's financial position continued to deteriorate, and there was a resurgence of support for the NDP. In the May 1986 election, the Conservatives took 60 of 83 seats in the legislature, but the NDP gained 15 seats, for a total of 17. The NDP won 29 per cent of the vote, almost double its best result in Alberta since the formation of the party (*Globe and Mail* 9 May 1986: 1). The government, aware that the NDP would be able to make considerable political capital of the extra-billing issue in the legislature and concerned to regain the funds being held by Ottawa, began to negotiate a settlement with the provincial medical association. Politicians were also eager to avoid a bitter dispute comparable to the one that was underway in Ontario (*Globe and Mail* 12 July 1986: A3). In August 1986, agreement was reached on a fee schedule acceptable to both the government and the profession, in return for an undertaking that extra-billing would be abolished.[29] Thus, two years after the Canada Health Act came into force, only New Brunswick still allowed doctors to extra-bill, but the practice was always very limited in that province.[30]

Hospital user-charges were never an issue of the same magnitude as physician extra-billing and became important mainly because of the Alberta proposals to introduce a 'universal system' of hospital charges. These plans were not implemented, and charges were eliminated in the province in 1986. Charges in Newfoundland were also abolished. The Ontario charge for long-term patients is not an infringement of the Canada Health Act. As in Australia, it is considered reasonable that people who reside permanently in nursing homes and other long-term institutions should contribute towards the cost of their 'lodgings.' The federal government withheld $13 million from Quebec up to the end of 1985 in respect of charges made to long-term rehabilitation patients. This charge was interpreted as an infringement of the conditions but is largely a definitional problem resulting from the need 'to fit the federal template over Quebec's very different system.' The problem has been exacerbated by the province's refusal to recognize the Canada Health Act. However, negotiations on the issue began at the end of 1985.[31] The important effect of the Canada Health Act regarding user-charges is that it is a disincentive to the use of this method of revenue-raising, since provincial treasuries no longer gain from the introduction of charges. Thus, the Canada Health Act has been almost entirely successful in preserving the universal system of public health insurance.

Conclusion

The governments of Canada achieved their major policy objective, which was to control the rate of increase in health-care expenditures, after the introduction of Medicare. In pursuing this politically risky policy, the critique of curative medicine that emerged in the 1970s was used to legitimize a limitation of resources allocated to therapeutic hospital and medical services. The division of responsibility for financing did not undermine cost-control measures, which were implemented by both levels of government.

The success of budgetary policy, however, gave rise to a number of political problems. First, expectations were created that resources would be diverted from traditional services and would be used to promote the expansion of primary-care and preventive health services. Second, the medical profession strongly opposed the cost-containment policies of both levels of government and charged that the health-care system was being underfunded. Pressure on physician incomes gave rise to an increase in the numbers of doctors charging patients an additional fee. In response, a wide range of groups mobilized, intent on achieving the preservation of the universal health-insurance system.

This array of pressures affected both levels of government. It is clear, however, that the division of responsibility offered the federal government a rare opportunity to gain political mileage without incurring heavy political costs. Despite provincial opposition, the Canada Health Act attracted very wide public support and, at the same time, placed the Conservative opposition in a no-win position. The federal government could be seen to be acting to preserve a popular national program without having to take responsibility for implementation. Moreover, as in the case of the Lalonde Report, the Canada Health Act cost the federal government very little. It was up to the provinces to find any additional money needed to reach settlements with provincial branches of the medical profession.

The provinces, for their part, were constrained by the national standards but, since there was strong public pressure to maintain the universal aspects of Medicare, provincial policy choices were limited, irrespective of the existence of the conditions. The government of Alberta postponed its plan to introduce a system of hospital fees before the passage of the Canada Health Act. It was reported in the press that this decision was a response to opinion-poll findings, although it may also have been partly a response to the announced federal determination to legislate. The federal division of responsibility acted as a valve through which pressures were relieved: it gave the provinces time to decide whether to take action to eliminate extra-billing and user-charges. Governments could have chosen to accept a reduction in federal funding rather than confront the medical profession. Moreover, there were three years in which to make the decision before federal funds were to be permanently withheld. So although the federal system gave rise to intense intergovernmental conflict, it also provided both levels of governments with a degree of flexibility not common in unitary systems. As more and more provinces legislated to outlaw extra-billing, the position of the medical profession became weaker and arguments that the standard of health care would deteriorate if extra-billing were eliminated became more difficult to sustain.

Had Canada been a unitary system, the same outcome might have been achieved by determined government action. The result, however, might have been a national doctors' strike, in which the government might have been defeated. It is more likely, however, that, faced with determined public pressure for action, a government would have proceeded by a number of incremental steps which is, in practice, what the federal division of power allowed. Federal legislation was followed by a series of provincial responses, staggered over time as political conditions changed.

In the early 1980s, most Canadian governments, including most members of the federal Cabinet, were not averse to a degree of reprivatization in the health-care system, especially if the effect would be to relieve budgetary pressures. The preservation of universal health insurance was not primarily a result of government initiatives. Rather, governments were pressed into action by public opinion, the NDP, organized labour, and other pro-Medicare groups. This pressure counterbalanced the political costs associated with opposition from the medical profession. Changes in public attitudes towards health and the health-care system appear to have been influenced by the critique of curative medicine. One doctor, writing in the CMA Journal about 'what went wrong,' argued that

the medical profession failed to anticipate that the public's awareness and knowledge of medicine could actually increase to the point where it threatened the physician's monopoly on his knowledge ... Many people have began to question the treatment given them, both medical and surgical. And it has become apparent ... that the basin of knowledge which was until recently proclaimed to be quite deep by the medical profession is in reality quite shallow ... Vocal spokesmen who are attempting to reimpose long-lost power and influence ... seem always to be waging a war which they have already lost. The physician must realize that he is no longer the total master of his destiny and that he cannot speak with absolute authority, especially in matters pertaining to health care delivery. (Richter 1986: 524)

Thus, just as public opinion pressured governments into action, it also assisted them in confrontations with the profession. The general decline in the authority of doctors appears to have been advanced further by federalism, which had given rise to a fragmented profession. The intense opposition of Ontario doctors to the Canada Health Act and to the provincial response was not shared by branches of the profession in provinces where extra-billing was absent or nearly absent. Combined with the enhanced opportunities for federal-government action, the flexibility afforded the provinces, and the 'demonstration' effect of Quebec Medicare, itself a result of the federal division of power, federalism appears to have been one of the factors that undermined the possibility of a united campaign against the abolition of extra-billing.

6

Compulsory Health Insurance in Australia, 1972–86

Between 1975 and 1984, there were *seven major changes* in health-insurance policy in Australia. This experience is patently at odds with claims that federalism obstructs change and/or gives rise to weak, conservative government. As discussed in chapter 4, most aspects of the voluntary insurance system came under intense scrutiny in the late 1960s. The scheme was criticized on grounds of equity, on the level of the premiums and the hardship this caused for many people, on the unpredictability of the share of costs borne by patients, and on the complexity and administrative expense of the scheme.

In the process of reviewing many of its policies, the Labor party adopted plans for a compulsory health-insurance scheme in 1969. The proposals became one of the major policies of the Whitlam government elected in 1972 and were implemented in 1975. However, the system was not secure from party political and professional attack and, in a series of piecemeal changes during the five years from 1976 to 1981, the Fraser non-Labor government completely dismantled the universal system in favour of a return to subsidized voluntary insurance.

The Labor party remained committed to universality and reinstated the original program, this time called Medicare, when back in office in 1984. Non-Labor is committed to reprivatization, a policy that should present few problems in view of the ascendancy of 'New Right' ideas in Australia unless there are changes in the level and intensity of public support for the national scheme.

This chapter traces the course of changes in the 1970s and 1980s and examines the factors that made such abrupt policy reversals possible. It is important to note that, in all cases, the main policy initiatives were taken by the Commonwealth. The role of the states was primarily reactive and, in many cases, they operated without any clear information about the Commonwealth's intentions. The centralization of power made it relatively easy for successive federal governments to impose their will on what is, essentially, a set of financial arrangements.

The Genesis of an Alternative Health Policy

In 1967, the leader of the opposition, Gough Whitlam, learned that the Hospitals Benefit Fund of Australia had bought an aeroplane to be used by management to visit branch offices. Interested in health policy and concerned that this might be an inappropriate use of contributors' money, Mr Whitlam asked his secretary, John Menadue, to find someone who understood the voluntary health-insurance system. Menadue contacted two economists, Dr J.S. Deeble and Dr R.B. Scotton, at the Institute of Applied Economic and Social Research, University of Melbourne. After discussion, a meeting was arranged between Whitlam, Deeble, Scotton, and several other people who were interested in health-policy reform. At the time, Deeble and Scotton's work consisted primarily of an analysis of the operation of the voluntary insurance system. They thought that compulsory insurance might rectify many of the problems of the voluntary system but had no concrete plans for such a scheme. During the next few months they developed proposals that were relayed to the leader of the opposition and to Labor member Dr Moss Cass, who had himself been working on plans for an alternative health policy. In April 1968, the outline for a compulsory-insurance system was completed. In the same month, Deeble and Scotton were invited to discuss their proposals with the Minister for Health, Dr A.J. Forbes, and with officials from the Commonwealth Department of Health. Because their scheme involved the abolition of the voluntary principle, it was rejected by the government (Freudenberg 1977: 102–5).

However, the principles of the plan were acceptable to Labor. In July 1968, in a speech delivered at the Royal Prince Alfred Hospital in Sydney, Mr Whitlam presented the proposals as 'The Alternative National Health Scheme.' This address was published in the *MJA* the following month and marked the beginning of an intense controversy, which remains unresolved more than twenty years later.

Compulsory health insurance, Deeble and Scotton argued, was 'the most efficient and rational way of combining both the insurance and subsidy functions of health cost pooling.' Unlike the situation in the United

States, where commercial insurance companies offered low-cost insurance to low-risk groups but where premiums for high-risk groups were prohibitively expensive, health insurance in Australia contained a subsidy element: the currently healthy subsidized the currently sick. Under voluntary insurance, this subsidization objective could be only imperfectly realized because many people in low-risk groups chose not to insure or to insure for low levels of coverage. Moreover, because of the 'accepted humanitarian principle that necessary services should not be denied because of inability to pay,' Scotton and Deeble argued that a health-insurance system should ideally provide for subsidization between high- and low-income groups. A system of flat-rate contributions could not achieve this objective. In order to overcome some of the problems of the system, separate arrangements had to be made for certain categories of people, such as pensioners, low-income earners, and the long-term and chronically ill. Scotton and Deeble argued that, while the voluntary system was improved by separate public subsidies for special groups, such was achieved only at the cost of greater complexity and expense. The result, they said, was neither 'voluntary' nor 'insurance.' Compulsory insurance, under which all who were 'deemed liable' were obliged to contribute and under which eligibility for benefits would be universal, provided a much simpler and more equitable solution.

The proposed scheme was to be administered by a statutory Commonwealth Health Insurance Commission. Revenue was to be raised by a levy of 1.25 per cent of taxable income, a matching Commonwealth subsidy, and a levy on worker's-compensation and third-party motor insurers. Income-tax concessions on net medical and hospital expenses and voluntary insurance contributions (for private hospital accommodation) were to be withdrawn. Benefits included coverage for medical costs and for standard public-ward care in public hospitals.

Doctors were to be paid on a fee-for-service basis for medical services except for services to patients in public wards of public hospitals, where remuneration was to be on a salaried or sessional basis. Doctors employed on a sessional basis contract to work a number of sessions (half-days) per week and are paid an hourly rate. There was to be a schedule of benefits for all services, based on 'standard' fees, which were to be determined by negotiation or arbitration. Doctors were not to be required to adhere to these fees and could, if they wished, bill the patient, who would then claim reimbursement from the commission. Alternatively, doctors could bulk-bill the commission at regular intervals and accept 85 per cent of the schedule fee as full settlement of their claims. The 15 per cent discount was calculated to be less than the cost of preparing accounts and of losses from concessional fees and bad debts. The proposal for bulk-billing was modelled directly on the scheme operating in Saskatchewan (Scotton and Deeble 1968: 9–16).

The Scotton–Deeble plan was adopted officially as the health policy of the Labor party at its federal conference in July 1969. The objective was to place 'comprehensive health care within everybody's reach' by means of an income-related tax and additional funding from general revenue. During Labor's long period in opposition, private medical practice on a fee-for-service basis had become institutionalized. A salaried medical service, which was still supported by some members of the Labor party, was rejected by Scotton and Deeble as politically unfeasible. However, elements from the era prior to insurance had survived in the hospital sector in Queensland and Tasmania, where private medical practice in hospitals was rare. The Queensland system served to demonstrate that it was cheaper to run a hospital system on the basis of fully paid medical staff. Free treatment in public wards of hospitals accorded with traditional Labor party policy, and it was planned to reintroduce this system on a national basis. The new policy could not guarantee that people would have access to free medical services but it was hoped that bulk-billing would become increasingly acceptable to the medical profession and that, through this mechanism, there would be no charge to patients at the point of service. Thus, by reintroducing the hospital policy of the 1940s and incorporating the Saskatchewan method of paying doctors, the prospect of access to free hospital and medical services could be offered.

The plans for compulsory health insurance dealt only with methods of paying for personal health services. The Labor party had also developed proposals for reform of the health-care delivery system through the establishment of community health centres and the relocation and upgrading of hospital facilities.[1] Taken together, the new insurance arrangements and the reorganization of the delivery system were designed to achieve an outcome that was consistent with Labor objectives first articulated in New South Wales in the early years of the century.

The Introduction of Compulsory Health Insurance

The Whitlam Labor government was elected to office in December 1972. The proposed insurance scheme, called Medibank, did not alter the private practice of medicine but rather changed the way in which people paid for insurance and received reimbursement. None the less, it was vehemently opposed by the medical profession. On the medical side, the main objection was to bulk-billing, which would automatically involve adherence to schedule fees. Doctors feared that if patients came to expect that they should not be required to pay part of the fee directly to the doctor, the system might eventually lead to the elimination of extra-billing.

The highly controversial hospital proposals were not a radical move but were 'a continuation of the system whereby services had been provided by an appointed staff of whom some were salaried and some worked on an honorary basis' (Sax 1984: 117). The main change was that all hospital medical staff were to be paid. The threat to the profession's interests was in the fact that because treatment would be available without charge, increasing numbers of people might choose standard ward care in public hospitals. Thus, although the system was unlikely to result in immediate changes, it had the long-term potential to reduce the size of the private medical market and to limit the freedom of doctors to set their own fees.

The possible expansion of the public hospital sector also posed a long-term threat to the viability of private hospitals, although the government offered substantial increases in subsidy rates. Moreover, the introduction of public health insurance meant that the functions of private insurance funds would be limited to providing coverage for private hospital accommodation and other services such as dental treatment, which were not included in the general arrangements.[2]

Compulsory insurance was therefore opposed by three main groups: doctors, private hospitals, and voluntary-insurance organizations. Between 1973 and 1975, these groups mounted an intense campaign of opposition against the government's proposals. They were strongly supported by the non-Labor parties, partly because the scheme was antithetical to Liberal ideology and partly because political capital could be made from the issue. The following selection of statements demonstrates the intensely ideological nature of the debate. Opposition spokesman for Health, Mr Chipp, speaking on the National Health Bill No. 2 in 1974, said 'if this Bill is passed by this Parliament, it will create a situation of anarchy in Australia. Anarchy is a situation not unknown to socialists. It is part of their bread and butter' (CPD HR, 3 December 1974: 4476). Traditional non-Labor concerns were expressed in a later debate on the same bill: 'the Bill which we are debating is a nationalistic, socialistic piece of legislation ... I am not interested in a socialised scheme or a nationalised scheme, but in a scheme that keeps free enterprise going in Australia' (Mr F.L. O'Keefe, CPD, HR 19 February 1975: 463–5).

The General Practitioner's Society (GPS), reporting to members, identified its main objections:

the intention of the Socialist Government is to extend the inadequate PMS [3] to every citizen of Australia and to coerce the medical profession into nationalisation ... the Government intends to use every possible measure to encourage patients to send unpaid accounts direct to the National Health Insurance Commission. This would enable the Commission to bulk-pay ... It is well known that he who pays the piper calls the tune ... By the same token, he who pays the money wields the stick. He who pays the doctor determines the quality and frequency of medical services and to some extent the place where the service is given. (*G.P. Society News* no. 1)

The manager of one of the largest voluntary insurance organizations, the Medical Benefits Fund of Australia, was of the opinion that 'some of our socialist economists and politicians want an income-tax-supported health service bought at the Government shop disguised as a Commonwealth Health Insurance Commission. Karl Marx's theories have never been wanted by Australians in the past, and they are needed even less today' (J.F. Cade, quoted in Sax 1984: 95). As in the 1940s, critics portrayed Labor policies as socialist or fascist schemes that would result in a loss of personal freedom. Cartoons put out by the GPS showed Labor leaders as Nazis, and patients tattooed with Medibank numbers.

The AMA had prepared and planned possible courses of action before Labor came to power. In 1973, it launched a publicity campaign of massive proportions. A public-relations firm was engaged, and advertisements were lodged in all sections of the media, including more than 250 television commercials per week. In 1973 alone, 16,000 publicity kits were issued for distribution. Doctors toured the country to address various community groups, and when it was felt that 'the public might be getting tired of hearing doctors,' the services of former Miss Australia, Sue Gallie, were engaged. In addition to the publicity campaign, 'a very active programme to inform and influence members of Parliament' was undertaken (AMA *Annual Report* 1973). Another part of the campaign included an aggressive stance on fee levels similar to that taken in the period of the previous non-Labor government (Sax 1984: 111–13). Some doctors resigned from the Pensioner Medical Service, and pensioners and other patients were circularized with the profession's views. The various branches of the AMA and the General Practitioners Society issued instructions to members and kept them informed. In New South Wales, 'territorial cells' were formed for the purpose of 'speedy communication, joint action and the protection of professional interests.' Members were advised to take an active part in the work of their regional cells.

Unlike the Chifley government, however, the Whitlam government did not need to reach an agreement with the profession in relation to medical services because no changes in the organization of practice were intended. After the necessary legislation was passed, the government needed only to provide an administrative structure for the payment of benefits and the collection of the levy before this part of the scheme could come into operation.

Mr W.G. Hayden[4] became Minister for Social Security in the new government. Mr Hayden had taken an interest in the health-insurance proposals and had developed considerable expertise in the area. It was decided that health insurance, dealing as it did only with financing arrangements, could appropriately be located in the Social Security portfolio, leaving the less controversial hospital and health-services policies with the Department of Health. Consequently, the medical- and hospitals-benefits divisions of the Department of Health were transferred to the Department of Social Security. One of the by-products of this move was a weakening of the well-established links that the AMA had with the department, thus reducing its influence at the bureaucratic level. However, the profession had been intensely critical of the plan for four years and under these circumstances the possibility of constructive discussions was remote (AMA 1969; AMA *Gazette* 21 September 1972).

Between 1973 and 1975, there were numerous meetings between the minister and the AMA, and between officials and the AMA, on the question of adjustment of schedule fee levels. There were fewer meetings, however, on the question of overall policy. An initial meeting with the minister in January 1973 was followed by two meetings with the minister's policy advisers and officials later in January and in February. In May 1973, the Health Insurance Planning Committee, chaired by Dr J.S. Deeble, tabled its report, known as the 'Green Paper.' The AMA and the other opponents of the scheme 'seized on the document to express their antipathy on numerous scores, some of substance, many more imaginary than real' (Sax 1984: 109). A detailed AMA submission on the report was made to the minister and was published under the title AMA *Views on the Deeble Plan* (June 1973). The government's proposals were 'totally rejected' on three broad grounds. First, there was 'no genuine community demand for change.' Second, the 'arbitrary imposition' of 'purely financial proposals' would place the work of the newly created Hospitals and Health

Services Commission in a 'strait-jacket.' Third, the AMA objected to 'the nature of the proposals,' which, it claimed, 'would lead to regimentation of the public, a lessening of free choice, a deterioration of health care standards by encouraging a uniform mediocrity. In the broad, the Committee's report is a blueprint for the rapid nationalisation of health care' (AMA 1973: 3).

Following this submission, the minister met with the royal colleges and the AMA and, in September, met again with the AMA. Discussions were formal, and no compromises were reached. A 'White Paper' was tabled in Parliament by the minister on 8 November 1973. Minor concessions were made including the elimination of incentives designed to increase the attractiveness of bulk-billing but there were no compromises on the principles of the proposed scheme.

In the meantime, the necessary legislation was in preparation, and the AMA concentrated its efforts on the parliamentary arena. Its objectives were 'defeat, amendment or delay of legislation by the Senate where the Government had no majority' (AMA Annual Report 1974: 14–15).

This strategy was initially successful. On 11 December the Health Insurance Commission Bill, 1973, and the Health Insurance Bill, 1973, were rejected by the Senate. Both bills were reintroduced in Parliament in April 1974 and were again rejected by the Senate. On the basis of the provisions of the constitution that deal with a deadlock between the House of Representatives and the Senate (Section 57), these bills (and four others) were used to call a simultaneous dissolution of both Houses of Parliament.

An election was held on 18 May 1974 at which the government was returned to power, but with a reduced majority in the House of Representatives and still without control of the Senate. Section 57 provides that if, after such a dissolution, the same legislation is again rejected by the Senate, a joint sitting of both Houses may be held. The legislation is deemed to have been passed by both Houses if affirmed by an absolute majority of the members sitting together. The Health Insurance Bill and the Health Insurance Commission Bill were passed at the first joint sitting of Parliament in Australia's history on 7 August 1974. Two bills relating to the imposition of a health-insurance levy did not meet the constitutional requirements of Section 57, so the government was forced to finance the scheme entirely from general revenue.

Realizing that there was now nothing to prevent the medical-insurance side of the policy from coming into operation on 1 July 1975, the federal president and other leaders of the AMA called on the minister in

August 1974 and informed him that Federal Council would no longer oppose the scheme. Future discussions should be held with the state branches.[5] In withdrawing its general opposition the AMA had effectively conceded the medical-insurance side of Medibank but the hospital program required negotiations with the states. In this process, AMA opposition was crucial.

Negotiating Hospital Cost-Sharing Agreements

Despite intense ideological opposition on the part of some members of some state governments and much rhetoric about 'states' rights,' the main obstacle to commonwealth–state agreement was the reluctance of three of the four non-Labor states to become embroiled in a confrontation with the medical profession about methods of paying doctors for hospital work.

The policy of the AMA was that remuneration should be on a fee-for-service basis for both public and private hospital patients. The Commonwealth agreed that fee-for-service payment would be continued for private patients but rejected the proposal for fee-for-service for public-patient medical services. The federal government pointed to the Nimmo Committee finding that the medical profession had already taken honorary work into account when determining the level of private medical fees. It was estimated that fee-for-service payment for the work performed in an honorary capacity would be three times as much as salaried and sessional (time-based) payment at generous levels. The government therefore proposed that the system operating in Queensland, in repatriation hospitals, and in the large teaching hospitals of some states should be adopted. It was argued that a system of salaried and sessional payment had operated successfully in Queensland for over thirty years and had the full support of that branch of the AMA. This proposal had been supported by state ministers for health, who, at the 1971 Australian Health Ministers' Conference, had adopted a resolution that, where the honorary system was to be replaced, a system of sessional payments for visiting specialists should be instituted. It was argued that this system would 'be in the interests of patient care and would provide better administration of hospitals and a better form of medical teaching.' In country areas, where the demand for certain services was too small to justify a specialist attending a hospital for a session, it was recognized that a modified form of fee-for-service might be an appropriate method of remuneration.[6]

Following the release of the Green Paper in May 1973 federal–state negotiations began at both ministerial and officer level on new financial arrangements for meeting hospital costs. The Commonwealth proposed a method of formula funding that was of greatest benefit to low-spending states. The highest priority from the state perspective was that the financing system should provide full protection against inflation, a concern that was understandable since the Commonwealth hospital benefit had not been increased since 1957. The Labor states that were negotiating seriously with the federal government argued that the formula proposed in the Green Paper did not guarantee this. They wanted the Commonwealth to meet a fixed proportion of expenditure, even though they would have gained more relative to three of the other four states under formula funding. Overall federal outlays were the same under both methods, and it was important for the government that the scheme begin as soon as possible in the Labor states. It was therefore agreed that a system of 50–50 sharing of net hospital operating costs would be adopted. These arrangements were set out in the White Paper released in November 1973.

Thus the main outlines, if not the details, of new federal–state financial arrangements were settled in 1973. After the rejection of the enabling legislation in the Senate, negotiations with the states were discontinued. Commonwealth officials and policy advisers turned their attention to devising alternative arrangements that might secure passage in the Second Chamber. In August 1974, following the passage of the necessary legislation at the joint sitting of Parliament, the prime minister wrote to the premiers, suggesting that discussions be resumed. The Minister for Social Security also wrote to the state health ministers. Examples of possible agreements were attached. Discussions at officer level were then held with Queensland, South Australia, and Tasmania. As no reaction, other than acknowledgment of letters, was received from the other three states, the prime minister again wrote to these premiers in December 1974. New South Wales and Western Australia replied with counter-proposals, which were unacceptable to the Commonwealth. The Minister for Social Security then wrote to the West Australian and New South Wales Health ministers. He suggested that discussions could be held about issues on which agreement might be reached. In a press statement on 12 March 1975, Mr Hayden announced that Western Australia had declined his invitation and that the New South Wales Health minister had postponed a meeting that had been scheduled for that day. No reply had been received from Victoria. Because of the delay caused by refusals to negotiate, the minister said that the Medibank hospital program would not be able to begin operation on 1 July 1975 in these three states.

In the meantime, satisfactory negotiations had been proceeding with the Labor governments of South Australia and Tasmania. In a joint press statement, the two Health ministers and Mr Hayden announced on 6 March that the full Medibank program would come into operation in these states on 1 July 1975 as planned.

At this time, the four non-Labor states were attempting to fashion a 'common front' to put before the Commonwealth. A meeting of state Health ministers was held on 4 March at the request of the premiers. Only the non-Labor ministers attended the afternoon session. After discussions with state officials, Dr R.B. Scotton, Chairman of the Health Insurance Commission, wrote to Mr Hayden, informing him that the meeting had been 'the occasion for some quite bitter politicking' and that 'despite the outward appearance of a common front' there was 'little trust between the States.' It was reported that the Queensland minister had denied having any firm offer from the Commonwealth, which the New South Wales minister did not believe. Health minister A.H. Scanlan of Victoria had 'categorically refused' to reveal his government's position. New South Wales is reported to have been of the opinion that Victoria was ready 'to do another last minute deal' with the Commonwealth and although the premier of Queensland was said to have contacted the premier of New South Wales, suggesting that they 'get together to defeat Medibank,' New South Wales thought that Queensland would soon enter an agreement. It was reported that 'very strong pressure' had been put on the New South Wales Health minister not to meet with Mr Hayden on 12 March.

The first positive response from Victoria in relation to negotiations was not received until 26 March 1975. Mr Scanlan, 'on behalf of the Health Ministers of Western Australia, Queensland and New South Wales,' invited Mr Hayden to a meeting to be held on 11 April, 'to discuss Medibank.' Mr Hayden accepted the invitation. The key issue in discussion was the states' proposal that doctors should be remunerated on a fee-for-service basis for medical services in public hospital wards. This was, of course, AMA policy. The meeting decided that the matter should be referred to officer-level discussions. The states requested that these discussions be on a multilateral basis but the Commonwealth insisted on bilateral negotiations. In a report to the prime minister, the Minister for Social Security expressed his opinion that New South Wales, Western Australia, and Victoria were sensitive to the political costs of remaining outside the program and were now 'quite keen' to proceed towards agreement.

There were strong financial incentives for the states to enter the program. As the target date of 1 July drew nearer, Western Australia, Victoria, and New South Wales became increasingly anxious to sign agreements. The Commonwealth, however, was not confident that these states could guarantee to provide medical services to public-hospital patients without charge. Moreover, in view of the serious budgetary problems that accompanied the onset of recession, the Commonwealth was rather less anxious to enter large cost-sharing programs than previously.[7]

Final Negotiations with the Non-Labor States

In Queensland the hospital system that the Commonwealth proposed was already in operation. The question was whether the state, for a variety of political reasons, would refuse to accept Commonwealth money.[8] The political forces at work were complex and involved both the premier's intense ideological opposition to the Commonwealth Labor government and its policies and an internal struggle between the parties of the ruling National–Liberal coalition. Financial considerations were complicated by the possibility that equalization arrangements might be upset if Queensland entered an agreement but New South Wales and Victoria did not. The treasurer, Sir Gordon Chalk (Liberal), had publicly announced that Queensland would enter the scheme, but Cabinet appears to have been divided on the issue. On 25 June 1975, the Minister for Health, Dr L.R. Edwards (Liberal), wrote to Mr Hayden, informing him that Cabinet had determined 'in principle' to enter an agreement. The matter was still undecided, however, on 11 August when the Queensland Health minister sent a telegram to Mr Hayden, requesting that a copy of the final agreement be forwarded immediately for further Cabinet consideration.[9] On 14 August the Queensland Cabinet authorized the premier to sign, and cost-sharing came into operation from 1 September 1975.

By far the most important issue in negotiations between Western Australia and the Commonwealth was the question of the terms and conditions relating to the appointment of medical staff in hospitals. After discussions at ministerial and officer level in April and May 1975, the premier wrote to the prime minister, expressing willingness to sign an agreement. The proposed agreement was rejected by the Commonwealth because clauses relating to the payment of doctors and the provision of diagnostic services in hospitals had been omitted. The details of methods of cost-control were also unacceptable. However, after lengthy discussions between officers, the Western Australian Health minister informed Mr Hayden on 13 June that 'considerable progress' had been made. Western Australia had been able to arrange for the medical staff of teaching hospitals to be paid on a salaried or sessional basis. No changes were required in the North West or in remote hospitals where doctors were already paid by salary. In peripheral metropolitan and country hospitals, however, doctors had previously charged medical fees to insured public patients and wanted these arrangements to continue. After negotiations, it was agreed that a modified fee-for-service system would be introduced. This system had been foreshadowed in the White Paper and was to operate in country hospitals in South Australia. Where salaried or sessional arrangements could not be negotiated, medical services would be provided on a contractual or modified fee-for-service basis. Under this system, hospitals contract with doctors to provide services for an agreed percentage of the schedule fee. The hospital, rather than the patient, pays the doctor. This arrangement was incorporated into the hospital agreement, along with the following clause: 'Western Australia will take appropriate action to ensure that a doctor agreeing to provide medical services to hospital patients on a salaried or sessional basis does not render an account to the patient.'

Negotiations between Victoria and the Commonwealth had been impeded by the fact that both the Minister for Health, A.H. Scanlan, and the Secretary of the Department of Health, G.W. Rogan, were intensely opposed to Labor policies on ideological grounds.[10] Bilateral negotiations were held with Commonwealth officers on 22 April 1975, and on 1 May, state and federal officials met with fourteen members of the Victorian branch of the AMA. 'Considerable progress' was reported to have been made at this meeting, but it was thought that the remaining problems would 'take several months to resolve.' Later in the month, the Victorian premier personally took charge of the negotiations.

At a meeting in Canberra with Mr Hayden and officials on 18 June, Premier Hamer announced that he was 'tired of the mutual attacks through the press' and was 'keen to have the situation resolved one way or another.' He said that he had studied the Tasmanian and South Australian agreements and 'could find little to object to.' He thought that the honorary system should be abolished but was not prepared to have it replaced with a fee-for-service system.[11] Apart from Mr Hamer's concern that the new system might lead to a shortage of public hospital beds if demand increased, the entire discussion centred upon anticipated difficulties with the medical profession. Towards the end of the meeting, Mr Hamer said that there were no differences at all between the two governments and gave an undertaking to keep any commitments that were made, with the proviso that Victoria would 'need a bit of flexibility.' Communications continued between Mr Hayden and Mr Hamer, and, in the meantime, medical staffing arrangements were negotiated on a hospital-by-hospital basis by Victorian officials. On 15 July, Mr Scanlan was able to provide a list of arrangements for the provision of medical services in all Victorian hospitals, which fully satisfied the Commonwealth's conditions. After further communications between Mr Hayden and Mr Hamer, in which Mr Hayden sought assurance that arrangements with medical staff could be finalized in the short time remaining, the scheme began operation in Victoria on 1 August 1975.

As in Queensland, differences of opinion within the government of New South Wales appear to have been a factor delaying Commonwealth–State agreement. In March 1975, the Health Commission of New South Wales was of the view that the cost-sharing offer was 'the best deal ever offered by an Australian Government' and the best ever likely to be offered, even though it might be 'a step in the direction of an inevitable Federal takeover.' The budgetary situation of New South Wales hospitals was described as 'disastrous.' The commission, with treasury support, is said to have argued strongly that the federal offer be accepted. The Minister for Health, Mr Healy, is reported to have been persuaded by these arguments.

As the West Australian and Victorian premiers had done, Premier Lewis wrote to the prime minister on 30 May, indicating his willingness to sign an agreement, but the terms were again unacceptable to the Commonwealth. On the same day, Mr Lewis issued a press statement, saying that New South Wales reserved the right to set fees for private patients and to determine the method of paying doctors. However, as 1 July approached, New South Wales urgently sought to sign an agreement. The Commonwealth was not convinced that sufficient agreement had been reached with the medical profession to enable the scheme to begin and suggested further discussions. Negotiations with the medical profession proceeded slowly, and in August were said to have reached an impasse. However, by the middle of September, doctors in teaching hospitals, some surgeons, and most physicians had agreed to accept sessional contracts. Modified fee-for-service was to be the basis for payment in country hospitals. Some groups of surgeons refused to accept sessional payment and continued as honoraries, but enough agreement had been reached to enable the scheme to operate. On 18 September, the New South Wales Health minister and the Commonwealth treasurer announced jointly that the Medibank hospital program would begin on 1 October 1975. On that date, only three months after the planned commencement, the complete Medibank scheme came into operation on a national basis.

The Determinants of State Responses

This account of federal–state negotiations between 1973 and 1975 clearly shows that the key obstacle to agreement was the reluctance of the three Liberal state governments to confront the medical profession. While ideological differences and party political factors were also important, the outstanding issue became whether agreement could be reached with doctors. The political cost of a lengthy dispute that might disrupt hospital services was a primary concern.

However, there were a number of factors that induced the states to 'cooperate.' First, the financial attractiveness of 50–50 cost-sharing helped to overcome objections. As shown in chapter 4, the Commonwealth share of hospital financing had fallen steadily after 1963, reaching a low of 13 per cent in 1974–5. In the first year of cost-sharing, the Commonwealth contribution rose to 40 per cent and the states' share fell from 55 to 37 per cent. Thus, while the medical profession saw the return of a non-Labor federal government as a solution to its problems, the states could have little confidence that this would assist them with the problems of hospital finances.

Second, Commonwealth policy presented the states with an opportunity to solve a long-standing difficulty in relation to the provision of hospital medical services. In the early 1970s, the medical profession had pressed for the abolition of the honorary system and for its replacement by a fee-for-service method of remuneration. The states had strongly resisted on grounds of cost. Officials had calculated that the provision of in-hospital medical services on a fee-for-service basis would cost four times as much as sessional, time-based payments. In 1972, the states combined together to request federal financial assistance to enable them to offer sessional remuneration to honorary staff. The Victorian premier adhered to this position in 1975. Medibank arrangements in relation to the payment of hospital doctors had been state policy for a number of years. Moreover, because costs were to be shared equally between the two levels of government, it was in the states' interests as much as that of the Commonwealth to limit the expansion of physician remuneration on a fee-for-service basis.

Finally, there were political pressures that induced the three states to enter the scheme. Once Tasmania and South Australia joined with Queensland in providing free public-hospital care, the Liberal states could be seen to be withholding benefits from citizens. The attempt to create a 'common front' against Canberra was partly a recognition that, if one of the three accepted the offer, the pressure on the other two to follow suit would be increased. In response to concern about adverse public opinion in June 1975, the Victorian government placed several large advertisements in the *Age* newspaper, assuring citizens that it had agreed to enter the scheme but was fighting for a better deal. Medibank was a very important program involving questions that needed serious consideration, the advertisements said. The Victorian government was 'working to make Medibank work better' (*Age* 9, 10, 11 June 1975). Thus, a combination of financial incentives and political pressures overcame the Liberal states' objections.

The process by which Medibank hospital arrangements were introduced was similar to the way health policies were implemented in Canada, although the states responded more quickly than most provinces. The evidence again suggests that federalism can operate to undermine rather than augment the influence of interest groups. As the pressure on the states increased, the medical professions' position became weaker. At the state level, officials were able to bypass local branches of the AMA where necessary, and negotiate directly with hospitals. While organized medicine opposed the scheme in principle, individual doctors gained by being paid for services that they had previously provided free. In different ways, in different states, doctors were persuaded to cooperate.

If the implementation of Medibank had depended upon the federal government reaching an agreement with the AMA, as in the 1940s, it would almost certainly have failed. The outcome of a meeting held at the end of 1974 is sufficient to illustrate this point. The Commonwealth had decided that it might be 'tactically useful' to approach the AMA to offer information about procedural matters and to discuss questions relating to bulk-billing arrangements and the provision of in-hospital medical services. The federal executive accepted an invitation to meet with Commonwealth officials.

On the appointed day, the president of the AMA declared the meeting open and then read the following statement: 'the purpose of the meeting this morning must be made clear. The AMA is in a position of direct confrontation over the government's proposal to introduce its health scheme on 1 July 1975, or at any other date. Consequently, this morning the AMA Executive is meeting the representatives of the Government to listen, but members will not be questioning or making comment on the information

provided by the government representatives.' As indicated in the statement, members did not discuss the issues or make comments. After officials had presented information on various aspects of the scheme, the
president of the AMA thanked them and closed the meeting. Clearly, the
prospect of agreement was remote in the extreme.

The states were far more successful than the Commonwealth in deal-
ings with the medical profession. They were experienced in running their
hospital systems and could negotiate arrangements at several levels, where
necessary. The introduction of Medibank, like the introduction of hospital and medical insurance and the elimination of extra-billing in Canada,
shows that a federal division of power can provide policy makers with a
high degree of flexibility. Policies do not need to be introduced nationally
on a given day. The political process can be worked out over a period of
time, and a variety of methods of dealing with opposing interest groups
can be utilized.

The main weapon in the Commonwealth's armoury was 'the power
of the purse.' But just as Labor used federal financial dominance to facilitate the introduction of Medibank, so non-Labor was able to use the same
power to dismantle the system.

The Fraser Period, 1976–82

Ten weeks after Medibank came into operation in all states, the Fraser
Liberal–Country party government was elected to office. One of its campaign planks was the promise of a 'new federalism' that would return
power to the states and reverse the overtly centralist approach of the
Whitlam government. Another was an undertaking to maintain Medibank. In the event, neither commitment was kept. The new federalism
turned out to be 'but a difference in the style of Commonwealth domination' (Sawer 1977: 8), of which the termination of Medibank was just one
aspect.

A Medibank Review Committee, composed of three senior Commonwealth officials, was appointed a month after the government came to
power. Members of the committee visited the states to obtain information, but there were no consultations about proposed policy changes.[12]
Medibank Mark II was announced in May 1976 as part of a mini-budget.[13]
The main features of the original scheme were retained but a levy of 2.5
per cent of taxable income was introduced.[14] Public insurance, however,
was no longer compulsory, and people could choose to 'opt out' and not
pay the levy if they took private insurance. The system was designed to

produce a '50–50 division of business between the public and private sectors and this was almost exactly achieved' (Deeble 1982b: 435). A very similar set of arrangements had been considered by Labor in the first half of 1974, when the Medibank legislation had been rejected in the Senate. Medibank Mark II reduced the Commonwealth deficit by an estimated $800 million but added 3.2 per cent to the consumer price index (CPI). Concessions to the medical profession added pressure to rising health-care costs (Gray 1984: 6).

As in Canada, the hospital cost-sharing agreements did not enable the federal government to control its share of expenditures. In May 1976, the Commonwealth declared the agreements invalid on grounds of a legal technicality, action that would be politically unthinkable in Canada. Hospital payments to all states were stopped immediately. Some states initially expressed the intention of taking court action to try to enforce the upholding of the agreements but, in the event, did not do so. The legal validity of the agreements was uncertain, but 'more importantly, the states' budgetary situations could have become intolerable while litigation proceeded' (Scotton 1980: 185). New arrangements were introduced, under which the Commonwealth met 50 per cent of 'approved' hospital budgets. A cumbersome procedure for determining approved costs was instituted that enabled Commonwealth officers 'who had seldom set foot in a hospital ... to challenge the decisions of their state colleagues' (Sax 1984: 136). The completely dominant position of the federal government was demonstrated in 1977 when it announced in the budget that its 'agreed' share of funding would be reduced by 5 per cent. The states were neither consulted nor were they given prior notice before the decision was announced (Sax 1984: 136; Scotton 1980: 185).

Health-care costs continued to rise and were reflected in higher insurance premiums. In response, calls were made for an increase in the levy to prevent a drift back to public insurance. The problem was that raising the levy to stabilize the shares of public and private insurance would increase the CPI and exacerbate the inflation rate. After a process of 'protracted agony' in which a multitude of schemes and changes were considered (Sax 1984: 155), health-insurance arrangements were changed twice in 1978. Free public-hospital care was maintained. A universal medical benefit of 40 per cent of the schedule fee was introduced. This benefit, of course, cut 60 per cent off the existing one. The levy was abolished and, with it, compulsory insurance, which reduced the CPI but increased Commonwealth expenditure. In 1979 the public subsidy for medical services was further reduced when the Commonwealth undertook to meet only costs in excess of $20 per service. The resulting saving for the federal treasury was an estimated $150 million per year. At the same time, rises in hospital charges for insured patients and in medical fees further increased the costs of private insurance (Sax 1984: 146–62). Thus the combination of cost and the protection offered by Commonwealth cover for expensive services induced people to become uninsured. Between March 1979 and March 1980, the number of people holding private insurance fell by 10 per cent (Deeble 1982a: 717).

Throughout 1979 and the first half of 1980, health policy attracted intense criticism from several provider groups. The viability of some private funds was threatened by the increasing proportion of high-risk contributors, and private hospitals and private medical practice were threatened by the fall in private insurance. Uninsured low-income earners no longer had cover for many medical services. The AMA issued a series of press statements, warning the government that health might well become an issue at the 1980 election, and the *Australian* declared health policy to be a 'total, unmitigated disaster' (29 October 1979). However, the government perceived that there was strong opposition to yet another policy change, and it was decided to delay action until after the election. An inquiry into the administration and efficiency of hospitals was set up, and a new federal Health minister undertook the task of negotiating with the AMA in an effort to prevent the organization from 'resorting to the press release.'[15] Health was thus successfully defused as an issue in the October 1980 election. The government was returned to power but it lost control of the Senate. However, new senators were not due to take their seats until July 1981 so that the government had eight months, during which time the passage of further legislation was assured.

In the first months of 1981, health again became a highly controversial issue. The report of the Commission of Enquiry into the Efficiency and Administration of Hospitals (1981) recommended that the cost-sharing agreements, which were due to expire later in the year, should be replaced by block grants on a per-capita basis. The AMA, aware of the importance of maintaining the federal share of funding, wanted cost-sharing replaced by special-purpose grants. The federal coordinating departments, however, advocated the absorption of hospital payments into general tax-sharing arrangements (Sax 1984: 168). So serious was the threat of a complete federal withdrawal from health policy that the AMA issued a press release condemning reports from 'unnamed government sources' that the Commonwealth Department of Health was about to be abolished (Press Release, 19 February 1981). In the first four months of 1981, Cabinet is reported to have spent more time discussing health than tax policy (*Canberra Times* 13 April 1981).

A new health policy was announced in April 1981. The remnants of Medibank were abolished. Commonwealth benefits were restricted to the privately insured, with special arrangements for pensioners, the poor, and those eligible for sickness benefits. Flat-rate insurance contributions were to attract a 30 per cent tax rebate at a cost to the Commonwealth treasury of $600 million per year in tax expenditures. Federal funds for hospitals and community-health and school dental services were absorbed into general revenue grants but remained temporarily 'identified,' a decision that represented a compromise between the AMA and the coordinating departments' positions. However, there was no requirement that the funds be spent on the services for which they had previously been allocated. While financial responsibility was returned to the states, there was no devolution of power. The Commonwealth determined that fees should be charged for all hospital inpatient and outpatient services, except for pensioners and those whom the federal government determined were disadvantaged. Federal funds were reduced by the amounts that the Commonwealth had calculated the states could raise through the reintroduction of hospital fees. The states were not consulted about the changes. As in 1952, fees were reintroduced in all states except Queensland, and Australia's second free hospital system was terminated (Sax 1984: 170; Mathews 1983: 40–1). Although the AMA view on federal funding arrangements did not prevail, the association 'warmly welcomed' the changes that it said were in line with its own proposals (AMA *Annual Report* 1981: 7–9). The voluntary health-insurance system designed by the medical profession in the late 1940s had been reinstated.

Several factors facilitated the termination process. First, unlike the Whitlam government, the Fraser government controlled the Senate. Second, powerful health-provider groups supported termination. Third, at a time of high inflation and high unemployment, the government was able to justify reprivatization on grounds that sound economic management required a reduction in the size of the public sector. Finally, the Medibank program had not been in operation long enough for people to come to rely upon it.

The termination process was not without difficulty, but the politics of federalism played a very minor role. The most serious problems arose from the incompatibility of the government's own objectives. On the one hand, the aims were to reduce Commonwealth expenditure, to reduce the size of the public-insurance sector, and to control escalating costs in order to maintain the attractiveness of private insurance. On the other hand, the Commonwealth wanted to control increases in the CPI as part of its drive against inflation and wage rises. However, privatization increased the CPI and weakened the government's capacity for cost control. The retention of an element of universality until 1981, in combination with rising premium levels, reduced the attractiveness of private insurance. The result was that a stable balance between the public and private parts of the program could not be maintained.

There was some political opposition to reprivatization but it was much weaker than opposition in Canada. The Australian Council of Trade Unions, the Australian Council of Social Services, the Doctor's Reform Society,[16] and the Labor party opposed termination. However, although the government pursued a cautious, incremental approach that was carefully orchestrated around election dates, political considerations were not sufficiently strong to force it to maintain the system (Gray 1984).

Thus Australian policy making contrasts strongly with the situation that led to the preservation and strengthening of the universal aspects of Canadian Medicare at about the same time. The states played a very small part in the whole process. From time to time, New South Wales politicians were critical of federal policies, but Labor was in power in only two states and, overall, little state-government comment was reported in the press. Compared with their Canadian counterparts, the states appear to accept federal domination as inevitable.

The Reintroduction of Universal Health Insurance

In February 1982, the Labor party launched what one newspaper called its 'big gun' for the 1983 election: the 'Hayden Health Plan' (*Sydney Morning Herald* 5 February 1982).[17] The proposal was almost identical with Medibank. Criticism and support followed well-established divisions, although a new argument was used by non-Labor and the AMA. The Labor proposals, it was said, would facilitate fraud by doctors (*Financial Review* 5 February 1982: 7; *Age* 5 February 1982: 3).

Labor returned to power in 1983. The new health scheme was named Medicare, and came into operation on 1 February 1984. The government did not control the Senate, but the Australian Democrats, who held the balance of power, decided, after considerable vacillation, to support the passage of the legislation. New hospital agreements were reached with the states with almost no difficulty. The only non-Labor governments were those of Tasmania and Queensland where the private sector of in-hospital medical practice was small. The National Party premier of Queensland repeated his familiar anti-Canberra, anti-socialist speeches, by which means he managed to persuade the prime minister to increase the compensation grant to his state by $35 million annually. Apart from the predominance of Labor governments at the state level, another important factor facilitated the introduction of the program: between 1975 and 1984, contract practice for hospital work had become established throughout the country, except in non-teaching hospitals in New South Wales. Thus, most governments did not face the prospect of a confrontation with the medical profession.

The commonly accepted federal depiction of the central government anxiously attempting to induce reluctant states to agree to its policies was reversed in this case. State Health ministers, who had assembled in Canberra in May 1983, had to wait for morning before discussions could begin because federal Cabinet had not made time to endorse the federal offer.[18] The absence of friction between the Commonwealth and the states in negotiating the new agreements is particularly surprising because the federal offer gave no financial benefits to the states. The financing system determined by the Fraser government was retained. The new agreements merely compensated the states for revenue lost when hospital fees were waived. Moreover, New South Wales could expect a confrontation with some of its doctors. Holmes and Sharman have argued that conflict 'simmers between the state and national levels of the parties.' They hold that this is partly 'an artefact of the existence of two levels of government' and partly 'a reflection of the differing policy preferences of the party activists based in their state party strongholds and those who hold party office at the national level' (1977: 114). In this case there was no evidence of 'simmering conflict' and, in the absence of financial incentives, the best explanation of the ready acceptance of the federal scheme appears to be the extent to which Labor policy is considered to be binding on all members of the party.

Thus, the introduction of Medicare contrasts with the introduction of Medibank in the relatively low levels of conflict surrounding the process. However, there were problems in New South Wales, where some specialists had opted to continue to work in an honorary capacity throughout the Fraser period, rather than be paid by hospitals. For this group of militant doctors, the introduction of Medicare meant that the number of hospital patients to which no fee could be charged would increase and the number of private patients in public hospitals would decline. Led by a group of 160 orthopaedic surgeons, New South Wales specialists began to resign their hospital appointments in what became a seventeen-month-long dispute. But the profession was not united, even in New South Wales, and only 40 per cent of specialists resigned. For most of the dispute, the AMA did not support the most militant organizations, the newly formed Australian Council of Procedural Specialists and the Australian Association of Surgeons. Attempts to extend the dispute to other states failed. The New South Wales government took a very hard line with the specialists and is reported to have been prepared to hold out longer than the Commonwealth before making concessions (Chesterman 1986: 79). Eventually, a settlement was negotiated. The federal government made five concessions, four of which were intended to increase the attractiveness of private hospital insurance. The fifth was the optional extension of modified fee-for-service arrangements to major country hospitals and peripheral metropolitan hospitals (Pensabene 1986: 76; Larkin 1989; Gray 1990). Although the settlement represented a minor gain for the medical profession, especially since the provisions apply to all states, it is not clear that the effects of the package will be as intended. The extension of modified fee-for-service decreases the attractiveness of private insurance because it enables patients to be treated by their own doctors in public wards rather than by hospital doctors (Chesterman 1986: 80). However, for the purposes of this study, the important point is that New South Wales supported the Commonwealth and, if anything, was prepared to make fewer concessions to the medical profession.

Conclusion

The Whitlam, Fraser, and Hawke federal governments were actively involved in making major changes in existing health-insurance arrangements. The centralization of financial power provided the Whitlam government with a means of influencing state policy and inducing state 'cooperation.' However, little was done to entrench Labor objectives because non-Labor was able to use the same power to terminate policies when it returned to office. Indeed, every change of government at the federal level since the 1940s has been followed by a major change in health policy. The capacity of the Commonwealth to alter policy almost at will has produced a great deal of confusion in the Australian electorate. This situation contrasts with the comparative policy stability in Canada, where policy changes have been preceded by protracted public debate. The combination of centralization and political polarization in Australia has resulted in much policy activity but very little policy 'development.' Australian experience supports Trudeau's (1968) argument that centralization may give rise to paternalistic approaches on behalf of government at the expense of democratic maturation in the electorate. In the confusion surrounding the many changes introduced by the Fraser government, up to 40 per cent of citizens were unable to decide whether they supported the new policies or not (Gray 1984: 13).

During the Whitlam period, the Senate was a serious obstacle to the passage of health legislation. The opposition was able to use its numbers to obstruct two essential pieces of legislation, which delayed the introduction of Medibank by a year. However, while bicameralism is a feature of Australian federalism, it is not an essential institution in a federal division of power. The Canadian Senate is an appointed body and does not have the same real power as its Australian counterpart. Powerful Second Chambers can be used to obstruct government action in unitary systems, and at both levels of government in federal systems. The crucial consideration is the perception of how such action will be viewed in the electorate.

The opposition of the four non-Labor states presented difficulties for the Whitlam government when Medibank was introduced. However, as the program commencement date drew near, it became clear that the Commonwealth was in a strong bargaining position as a result of its financial power. This strength was augmented by political pressure on the states to enter the program. Moreover, the states undertook the unenviable task of negotiating hospital arrangements with local branches of the medical profession and, in this, were able to achieve an outcome that met Commonwealth policy requirements. As in the case of the Canada Health Act, state opposition was perhaps a small price to pay for the benefit that accrued to the federal government when it did not need to negotiate a settlement with the medical profession.

The Fraser period clearly shows the power which the Commonwealth can exercise by reason of its financial dominance. Radical changes in hospital-financing policy were introduced without consultation with the states. This situation demonstrates the wide difference between the Canadian and Australian federations. The change from cost-sharing to block funding was 'negotiated,' although there was concern that the federal government would take unilateral action if agreements were not reached in Canada. The federal government conceded tax points to the rich provinces and better equalization arrangements to the poorer provinces. In Australia, the federal government did not consult with the states at all when instituting a similar policy change. Federal-provincial conflict in Canada is generally viewed negatively, and unilateral action of the kind taken by the Fraser government when declaring the hospital agreements invalid, or, in 1981, when the decision was taken to replace cost-sharing with general-revenue grants, would be tantamount to political suicide.

The centralization of power in Australia, at least in relation to health policy, thus gives the Commonwealth a level of policy freedom of a similar order to that found in unitary systems. While the 'revisionist' theory of federalism is a useful tool in explaining Canadian developments, it has little applicability in Australia. The states have had almost no independent impact on the main contours of policy since the 1940s, and the experience of the Whitlam and Fraser periods demonstrated that even their capacity to challenge Commonwealth initiatives is weak. Cries of 'States' Rights' during the Whitlam period did not evoke enough public support to deflect the Commonwealth from its course, and the Fraser period shows that the federal government can determine policy for state hospitals without the need even for consultation. Clearly, the institutions and politics of federalism in Canada and Australia are entirely different, and generalizations about the two federations can be made only in the broadest terms.

Finally, the introduction of Medicare in 1984 shows that federal–state relations are not always fraught with conflict and that there is not necessarily tension between state and federal politicians of the same party. The dominance of non-Labor at the state government level during the Fraser period, too, partly accounts for the relatively low level of state political reaction to unilateral federal decisions. In Australia, and to a much lesser extent in Canada, party political differences do increase intergovernmental tensions and reduce the likelihood that policy agreement will be reached. But intergovernmental conflicts can be played out only as far as electoral considerations allow. The Alberta government, as we saw in the last chapter, did not act on its plans to reprivatize health-insurance arrangements in 1983, and the Victorian government was keenly aware of the political costs of remaining outside Medibank in 1975. It needs to be shown, rather than assumed, that party or intergovernmental competition within a federation gives rise to policy outcomes that are substantially different from those that emerge in a unitary system or in a federation where one level of government is primarily responsible for policy. We saw in chapters 2 and 3 that, in some states and provinces, there was a clash of political forces when the policy environment resembled a unitary situation because federal governments were not involved. British Columbia and New South Wales both failed to implement most or all of their policies in the face of physician opposition, and Saskatchewan Medicare, as it was finally introduced, was far removed from the government's preferred policy. We saw, also, that the unitary governments of Britain and New Zealand failed to achieve many of their objectives in the 1940s. Thus the channelling of the same political forces through an extra level of government does not necessarily result in policy immobilism. Both levels of government in a federation are, after all, subject to many common political pressures. Under some circumstances, deadlocks and delays may occur but, under others, a division of power and responsibility can be used to cushion and defuse the impact of political opposition, as in the case of the Canada Health Act or the Whitlam government's Medibank.

7

Health Services in Canada and Australia, 1970–86

National health insurance is a means of financing personal medical services. It does not impinge directly on the organization of the health-care delivery system but rather provides financial underpinning for a set of pre-existing services. Some expansion of medical and hospital services may be promoted in low-income areas when financial barriers to access are removed but, by and large, the health-care delivery system remains unchanged. Hospital services continue to be provided, as under previous arrangements, and doctors remain free to determine what medical services to provide and where to locate their practices. Unless the definition of insured services is expanded, financial barriers to access to services provided by non-physican health professionals, such as nurses and counsellors, remain.

Relatively little attention was given to the health-care delivery system in Canada until after the introduction of national health insurance. However, in the 1970s, partly in response to concerns about cost control, a new set of ideas emerged about health and what should constitute health policy. It was realized that health insurance provided a solution only to the problem of paying for curative medical services. Through systems of health insurance, the overwhelming proportion of public funds was devoted to the treatment of episodes of illness. Critics argued that much of this illness was preventable, that the system promoted institutional care at the expense of domiciliary and community-based services, that areas such as occupational health and rehabilitation were neglected, and that services for groups such as the aged, the chronically and mentally ill, and the disabled were inadequate. The ideology of curative medicine – that illness and health are determined mainly by biological factors and that more health is the same thing as more medical services – began to be questioned. Many people argued that what had been euphemistically called 'health policy' was really illness policy, and then very narrowly defined. Other criticisms pointed out that the subsidization of privately produced medical services had not radically altered the serious maldistribution of services between high- and low-income areas and between city and country. Nor had it rectified the problem that some areas of medicine were oversupplied with qualified physicians whereas serious shortages remained in others. Moreover, the doctor-dominated, technologically oriented curative services fostered by insurance are expensive. It was widely argued that resources should be reallocated towards preventive and primary-care services provided by teams of health professionals based at the community level. The provision of such services would not only move the focus of policy away from illness and towards health but could also be a means of redistributing services geographically and between groups. Community care, it was argued, could be provided more cheaply than acute care and held the potential to greatly improve the health of the population.

Whereas concern about the health-care delivery system did not develop in Canada until after the introduction of national health insurance, the situation in Australia was quite different. Probably because of the strong Australian tradition of direct service provision, the Whitlam Labor government's reform package included intervention in the organization of the delivery system and an expansion of direct services, as well as national health insurance. Planning on a regional basis was to be undertaken in order to provide an integrated system of hospital, community-health, domiciliary, and related welfare services. A network of community health centres was to be established to provide extensive educational, preventive, early-detection, and rehabilitation services in addition to conventional diagnosis and treatment. Aboriginal health was to be given high priority. The school dental scheme was to be expanded to provide free treatment for all children up to the age of fifteen years. Other areas of concern included health 'manpower' planning and training and expansion of research (Everingham 1974: 16–26).

Most of these ideas were not new. The Australian states had long been involved in the direct provision of services not generally provided by doctors, and the federal government had attempted to set up health centres in the 1940s. Australian developments fitted in with proposals made in other countries: the establishment of health centres was first recommended in New York in 1919, and in Britain in 1920. New York centres were intended to overcome the problems arising from maldistribution of services and were to incorporate school medical, nursing, public-health, and education services and to provide treatment for communicable diseases. Maternal, child-health, diagnostic, laboratory, and general medical services were to be provided. The necessary legislation was passed in 1923, but implementation was prevented by the opposition of the medical profession. It was not until the late 1960s that centres along these lines were established in the United States with federal financial assistance. Neighbourhood health centres are located in low-income areas that are unable to support private medical practice. They provide valuable services to citizens but present no threat to the size of the medical market. In Britain it was only in the 1960s that health centres in which services are provided by teams of health professionals were established. Since then, the number of centres has increased, but the medical profession has been slow to accept the changes. Despite financial incentives, only 24 per cent of Britain's general practitioners worked in the centres in 1984 (Andersen 1984: 6–7).

Planning of the health-care delivery system and the direct provision of services is constrained by medical opposition. Government intervention in the delivery system poses a far greater threat to the financial and professional autonomy of private practitioners than does the introduction of health insurance. For this reason, proposals for a national network of community health centres were regarded by some as the more radical part of the Whitlam government's policy package (*Age* 20 June 1976).

In addition to medical opposition, other constraints, discussed in chapter 5, surround attempts to reform the health system. Briefly, these include the uncertain political and budgetary costs of new and untried programs, the absence of immediately identifiable benefits, and the possible disruption of existing services. The benefits of preventive health services are not readily apparent and are unlikely to attract wide public support in the short term. The acceptance of alternative services depends upon attitudinal changes on the part of both health-care consumers and health-care providers. Because opposition from providers is likely to be intense and because changes cannot be achieved quickly, successful reform requires strong political will over an extended period of time.

Despite these constraints, reforms were introduced in Canada and Australia after 1970, but followed very different patterns. Innovations reflect both the policy preferences of governments in office in different jurisdictions and the different distributions of power in the two federations. The decentralized nature of Canadian federalism and the relative fiscal autonomy of the provinces allow provincial experimentation. One province,

Quebec, undertook a radical reorganization of its health-care delivery system. In Australia, where the states are far more dependent financially, new health services and facilities were developed at the instigation of the Commonwealth during the period of Labor government between 1972 and 1975. The reforms were not nearly as comprehensive as those of Quebec but, because the federal government was at the helm, they extended to all jurisdictions. The evidence suggests that there is a trade-off between centralization with relatively uniform policy development and decentralization, which can lead to radical innovation in some jurisdictions and inaction in others.

Health Services in Quebec

As discussed in the previous chapter, both the federal and provincial governments used the critique of curative medicine in the 1970s to justify reduced expenditure on conventional health services. Little was done, however, to promote the development of alternative services or to develop a policy based on a wider social view of health. In contrast with other provinces, the political, social, and cultural situation in Quebec provided a unique opportunity for policy innovation. As in Saskatchewan in the 1930s, there were widespread demands for radical change.

Between 1944 and 1960, the province of Quebec had been governed by the Union Nationale Party. Backed by the church and the traditional middle class, these governments were 'rigid,' 'regressive,' and 'centralist' (Lee 1979: 3). Economic changes had transformed the society of the province from predominantly rural to urbanized and industrialized. The education system was dominated by the church and geared towards the provision of a classical education, which was unsuited to the needs of the new urban working classes (Coleman 1984). Economic domination by anglophone Canadians and Americans generated discontent among the francophone business class, and economic instability created insecurity for the working classes (Milner 1984: 269). Traditional institutions had been increasingly unable to cope with the changes in society, and the new urban working classes saw the church as increasingly irrelevant to their lives. Analysts disagree about the composition of the groups demanding change (Coleman 1984: 3–25), but there is no doubt that, by 1960, strong, broad-based support for fundamental economic, social, and political reform had emerged (Milner 1984: 268–75, Coleman 1984). The election of a revitalized Liberal party in 1960 ushered in a period of change known as the 'Quiet Revolution.'

Between 1960 and 1966, major economic, educational, and social reforms were introduced, and an organized and radically militant labour movement emerged. The education system was secularized, the first legislation to take control of the hospital system was introduced, and the power industry was nationalized. At this time, the Quebec government began to demand that Ottawa withdraw from conditional-grants programs so that the province could raise its own taxes and design its own social-welfare system.[1] These demands were supported by nationalist groups, which included sections of the middle classes, and by the province's three giant unions – labour, teachers, and farmers. As mentioned in chapter 2, a commission of enquiry under the chairmanship of Claude Castonguay was established in 1967 to study and make recommendations for the whole health-and-welfare system of the province.

Proposals for a New Delivery System

The Castonguay Report, which took six years to complete, comprises seven volumes and twenty-eight separately published appendices.[2] During the course of its investigations, the commission established many research projects, drew upon the experience of other provinces and countries, and held extensive public hearings. In order to gain information about the attitudes of disadvantaged groups, a number of public advisory committees were established (Lee 1979: 7).

Volume IV of the commission's report, released in 1970, contains recommendations for a complete reorganization of the health-care delivery system. The commission recommended that a coherent and integrated health system be established, to provide geographic, financial, and psychosocial access to comprehensive and continuous services. The health system was to be regionalized and decentralized. Each region was to have a health council with autonomous legal status and wide powers to plan and provide a complete range of services within its area. Hospitals were to absorb existing public-health units and were to be responsible for the provision of preventive as well as treatment services. New community-based centres were to be established, to be linked to hospital centres. Local health centres staffed by health teams were to provide for services for defined populations. Each region was to have at least one university health centre that would concentrate on the development and provision of highly specialized services (Castonguay 1975: 99–103; Lee 1979: 7–10). There was to be public participation at every level of the new system. No new acute-care hospitals were to be established. The commission recommended that the fee-for-service method of remuneration for physicians be gradually replaced by salary or case-based payments. Because of the experimental nature of the proposals, it was envisaged that heavy emphasis would need to be placed on evaluation (Lee 1979: 11–13).

The ideological tenets underlying the commission's proposals have been summarized by Gosselin (1985: 74) as follows:

1 Health issues were to be considered from a physical, mental and social point of view. Thus beyond the usual biological aspects, other major health determinants had to be considered by analysts and decision-makers, namely, environmental, sociocultural and behavioural.
2 Hospitals were encouraged (a) to gradually abandon the traditional, closed (medical) model and to adopt a more open (social) model, and (b) to focus on preventive programs as well as curative programs. All of this would ostensibly be accomplished through the intensive involvement of local people, including health care managers and professionals, citizen's groups and associations and other community representatives.
3 Health care was to be delivered through a variety of establishments, each having a specified role and all closely integrated with one another both horizontally and hierarchically. Health care would thus evolve into an interlocking system culminating at a central control point.

The Liberal party was re-elected to office in 1970 and immediately set about implementing the recommendations of the Castonguay Report. Another set of unusual circumstances greatly assisted the introduction of the changes. At the 1970 election, Claude Castonguay had been elected to Parliament and became Minister for Health and for Family and Social Welfare. At the same time, several members of the commission's staff were appointed to key positions in the bureaucracy. The result was that a group of researchers became responsible for the implementation of their own recommendations.

After the introduction of Medicare, reorganization began. The Department of Health was merged with the Department of Family and Social Welfare in 1971, to become the Ministry of Social Affairs. Its responsibilities were health services, social services, and income security.[3] Early attention was given to policies relating to physical and human resources. Almost all projects for the expansion of acute-care hospital facilities were cancelled. The construction of new facilities such as outpatient clinics, emergency hospital services, long-term care institutions, and local community health centres was begun after consultation with a wide range of groups. The main objective was to adapt resources to regional needs. An extensive review of training for health professionals was undertaken in collaboration with the relevant educational institutions. Global budgeting for hospitals was introduced, and hospitals were then free, within broad guidelines, to determine the use of allotted resources (Castonguay 1975: 102–7).

An Act Respecting Health Services and Social Services (Bill 65) was passed at the end of 1971. The act explicitly proclaims the right of every person 'to receive adequate, continuous personal health and social services from a scientific, human and social standpoint' and prohibits discrimination on grounds of race, colour, sex, religion, language, national extraction, social origin, customs, or political convictions. The broad social approach and comprehensive objectives set out in the legislation show the distinctive attitudes of Quebec policy makers at the time and contrast with the more limited aims of governments in other Canadian jurisdictions that focused on short-term cost-containment measures.

The Organization of Quebec Health Services

Bill 65 followed the recommendations of the Castonguay Commission in most important respects. One major departure was in the degree of autonomy given to the regional councils. Whereas the commission had recommended that wide powers be delegated to these bodies, the government was initially reluctant to relinquish central control so that the new organizations bore little resemblance to those envisaged by the planners. Although the legislation provided for the different institutions that would make up the system and set out the functions of these bodies, it made no attempt to determine the way integration would be achieved or to set out the linkages between the parts of the system. A third important change was that separate university health centres were not established. Instead, this function was devolved upon specified hospital centres (Lee 1979: 23–8).

Apart from the twelve regional councils, the other key institutions of the new system are local community health centres, social-service centres, reception centres, and departments of community health. Social-service centres provide services to hospital and ambulatory patients and citizens generally. Community health centres provide a comprehensive range of primary-care and preventive health services and social services.

Reception centres provide institutional-care facilities and rehabilitation services.

Thirty-two departments of community health (Les départements de Santé communautaire [DSC]) have been located in major hospitals throughout the province. These institutions are concerned with the development of preventive and public-health programs. The health needs of each territory are identified by epidemiological and public-health research. The departments are responsible for developing and implementing specific programs, for coordinating community efforts aimed at achieving specific health objectives, and for the evaluation of programs. DSC's work in cooperation with local community health centres (Les centres locaux des services communautaires [CLSC]) in developing programs in response to particular problems found in local areas (Pineault 1984: 93).

Implementation Difficulties

In view of the magnitude of the proposed changes, it is not surprising that policy makers initially encountered serious difficulties. Opposition emerged from many quarters. The medical profession was strongly opposed to the creation of CLSCs, in which there was to be community participation and where doctors were to be paid by salary. Reduced emphasis on acute-care facilities created antagonisms. A policy to convert 10 per cent of these facilities to long-term care units, which were in short supply, led to confusion and disruption. The government's reluctance to delegate responsibility to regional councils resulted in a heavy workload that the ministry could not handle satisfactorily. There were particular problems associated with the development of CLSCs. Within the ministry, administration of the program changed hands several times. Community organization was slow to emerge. The centres provided a base from which groups committed to social action criticized the government, and several centres 'exploded from the activities of competing internal forces, with differing perceptions of what the objectives were to be and how they were to be reached' (Lee 1979: 2). By 1975, the wisdom of establishing the seventy-one proposed CLSCs was being reconsidered. There were problems, too, in relation to the allocation of responsibility for the provision of services between different organizations, particularly as CLSCs were slow to become established.[4]

While many of the early problems were overcome by the mid-1980s, some of the aims of the commission had not been realized. One of the

least successful aspects of the policy was the attempt to integrate curative and preventive services. It was hoped that this would be achieved
by locating DSCs in large hospitals. However, hospital workers found that
preventive and public-health programs have little relevance to their functions. In some cases, there was conflict between DSCs and their hospitals
and, in others, the DSC was ignored by the rest of hospital staff (Pineault
1984: 94). In respect to their own functions, however, DSCs now operate
much as the planners intended (Trent 1984: 1187).

Efforts to promote community involvement have been partly successful. Over the years, the government gradually transferred responsibility
for planning and developing many services to the regional health councils. In 1981, responsibilities in relation to cost-containment were devolved
but the ministry retains the final say in relation to financing decisions
(Gosselin 1984: 10–26). Community participation at the primary-care level,
where the institutions are small and the concerns are local, has been successful. Here preventive-health programs reflect lay opinion about the
factors that constitute health and social problems (Pineault 1984: 96). However, at the secondary- and tertiary-care levels, there has been conflict
about resource allocation and disagreement about the types of services
that should be developed. According to one observer, 'patients needs continue to be defined in the organization's own terms and the services to
be offered from the organization's own perspective' (Gosselin 1984: 22).

Despite these shortcomings, in the opinion of former deputy minister
Dr Jacques Brunet, now executive director of the Hospital Centre, Laval
University, the system is working much as the Castonguay Commission
envisaged. Most of the planned facilities have now been established, and
the principles, priorities, and objectives established by the commission
have been maintained. He considers that the system is very dynamic because it is organized to allow for experimentation and innovation, particularly in the field of community health. Dr Brunet stresses that the changes
are ongoing and that the reorientation of the system is a very long-term
project.[5]

The Achievements of the Quebec Reforms

Health services in Quebec have been redistributed to provide greater accessibility and resources have been reallocated towards primary and preventive services. In 1979, there were fewer short-term and more long-term
beds than in any other province (Breau Report 1981: 100). Facilities have

been established in previously undersupplied areas, particularly through the creation of CLSCs. At the end of 1985, 135 community centres were in operation, and another 36 in the planning stages were expected to be in operation by 1987.[6] An unanticipated consequence of the CLSC project was that it promoted the reorganization and relocation of private medical services. The Federation of General Practitioners (FMOQ) regarded CLSCs as a threat to private practice. It urged its members not to join as salaried practitioners and mounted a campaign to promote the development of group practice polyclinics, which would provide services on a twenty-four-hour, seven-day-a-week basis, especially in areas where there was a shortage of doctors. This campaign was successful. About 400 polyclinics were established, resulting in a far better distribution of doctors (Lee 1979: 26). A more limited effort by the Society of Specialists (FMSQ) met with less success. Similarly, government policies in the form of financial incentives intended to provide a better distribution of specialists have failed to make much impact.

One of the most successful aspects of the Quebec reforms is the expansion of primary-care services. The proportion of general practitioners, which had been declining rapidly, was increased from 43 per cent of all physicians in 1972 to 48.5 per cent in 1981, and was expected to reach 51.8 per cent in 1986 (Trent 1984: 1188). This change has been brought about through the control of hospital training posts and by adjustments of the fee schedule to raise the status of general practitioners.[7] The objective is to achieve a ratio of general practitioners to specialists of 60: 40 by 1990 (Pineault, Contandriopoulos, and Fournier 1985: 421).

Community medicine has been established as a new specialty, which has done much to reverse a situation where publicly employed, public-health doctors held a low status within the medical profession. Several universities now offer training programs, and the results are reported to be spectacular. Young physicians are being attracted to the area, and graduates find posts in DSCS and CLSCs, on a salaried basis. Remuneration is attractive, prestige is high, and work within the centres is said to be rewarding and challenging, offering opportunities for innovation and experimentation in the fields of prevention and health promotion (Trent 1984: 1189; Pineault 1984).

After a shaky beginning, CLSCs are an established and expanding element of the health and social-services system. Because of initial difficulties in attracting doctors, CLSCs have not become the main institutions for the delivery of primary medical services, as was intended. However, there are indications that doctors' attitudes are changing, a development that will accelerate as the number of newly trained general practitioners increases. A survey undertaken in 1981 showed considerable changes in physicians' attitudes towards methods of remuneration. Two-thirds of the doctors surveyed expressed a willingness to change from fee-for-service to time-based payment, provided their incomes did not fall (Pineault, Contandriopoulos, and Fournier 1985: 419–30). CLSCs employed about 10 per cent of Quebec doctors in 1985.

The CLSC is an autonomous body, run by an elected board. Within its allotted budget, each centre is free to develop its own programs according to perceived local needs. There is thus a considerable variation among centres: some provide a wide range of services and have developed innovative programs; others have not. CLSCs are responsible for the delivery of both health and social services. It is in these centres that attempts are made to integrate prevention, treatment, and rehabilitation services. In some cases, the health function is the more important; in others, emphasis is on social welfare; elsewhere, preventive, educational, and counselling services predominate. About 500 community-action workers are employed throughout the province. The role of these workers is to deal with problems discovered in cooperation with other agencies such as Youth Protection, legal aid, and, sometimes, the police. Each CLSC is responsible for the population of a defined geographical area, and most have outreach programs that attempt to make contact with all vulnerable groups such as low-income families and aged citizens within the area.[8]

An understanding of the extent to which the community-centre method of service delivery differs from the traditional method of private-practitioner services can be gained by examining more closely the work of a local centre. CLSC Metro Guy in downtown Montreal is one of the largest and most successful centres.[9] Its client population includes wealthy and poor people, students, people who work in the city but live out of the area, and a high proportion of aged citizens. The centre runs a youth and women's clinic, a family life education project, a family therapy service, and a Home Care Program. Depending upon the problems found in the area, and according to client's requests, different programs are developed. In all undertakings, there is stress on prevention and education.

The Youth and Women's Clinic runs a wide range of programs designed to promote understanding of disorders and problems, as well as providing conventional services. The perinatality unit works closely with day-care centres in the area and runs educational, child-safety, pre- and post-natal, and child-health programs. The Family Therapy unit is responsible for counselling, whereas the Family Life Education program concentrates on education and problem prevention. Classes are run on a diverse range of topics, from step-parenting to ageing.

It is perhaps in the Home Care Program that the Castonguay Commission's objective of making a complete range of health and social services 'accessible to every person continuously and throughout his/her lifetime' is most fully realized. This program has attracted province-wide and international attention. With a staff of 26, assisted by 200 trained volunteers, 950 elderly people are maintained at home and provided with the services they need. Efforts are made to contact all aged persons in the Metro area, with the help of information from Statistics Canada. Nursing, advocacy, and long-term placement services are available, and household help is provided, as necessary. Seniors are brought to the centre regularly to attend various clinics and to participate in social activities. Emphasis is placed on rehabilitation and physical therapy, with the aim of maintaining or regaining self-reliance. Metro seniors carry identification cards so that the centre can be contacted in case of misadventure. The skills of the physically able are used in various aspects of CLSC work, where appropriate. Those who can afford to pay for services are encouraged to do so, but the centre locates the helpers, provides training if necessary, and coordinates the action. Information is available about rights of citizens and about changes in government policy that may effect seniors. Clearly, a program providing such a comprehensive and continuous range of services is highly innovative in the Canadian and Australian contexts. The CLSC movement demonstrates the radical changes in concepts of health care that have taken place in Quebec since the 1960s when a health service basically meant a treatment service delivered in the office of a private medical practitioner.

Quebec policy makers are quick to point out that not all CLSCs have developed a set of programs and services as comprehensive as those of CLSC Metro, which is something of a demonstration project. Decentralization, as Canadian experience so amply demonstrates, provides opportunities for innovation and experimentation, which, by definition, will result in uneven development of services and policies. Whether the objectives of reformers are more likely to be achieved under centralization or decentralization must remain an open question. A very large number of case-studies would be needed from which to try to generalize and even then the interaction of many complex factors, which would vary from issue to issue and from place to place, makes comparative evaluation somewhat hazardous.

Towards a 'Real' Health Policy

For decades, health policy in Western countries has focused upon providing access to medical services for sick people. Many of the Quebec reforms fall within this tradition. The geographical redistribution of services, the reallocation of resources to neglected areas such as rehabilitation, community health, and domiciliary care, and the use of non-medical health professionals are policies aimed to achieve 'medical care' objectives. Analysts have argued recently that 'health' objectives should be identified so that policy decisions might be made with reference to their impact on health rather than sickness. In this way, a 'real' health policy might be developed (Pineault, Contandriopoulos, and Lessard 1985).

While critical of the rate of progress, Pineault, Contandriopoulos, and Lessard (1985) acknowledge that some health objectives have been established in Quebec.[10] In the field of perinatal care, specific policies were instituted in 1973 designed to reduce the maternal and infant mortality rates and the incidence of premature birth, and, in 1977, a nutrition policy was launched. Planners have given attention to the care of the aged, aimed at increasing their autonomy. Other programs have promoted preventive dentistry, awareness of alcohol and tobacco abuse, and the need for physical exercise (Pineault, Contandriopoulos, and Lessard 1985). In addition to these centrally planned objectives, DSCs and CLSCs have been engaged in devising programs to meet locally determined health objectives. In the research field, resources have been channelled and directed towards identified problem areas. The Medical Research Council of Quebec decided that, at a time of economic restraint, adequate coverage of all aspects of research could not be achieved. Therefore, efforts are concentrated in specified fields. In 1985, epidemiology, mental health, and biotechnology were being given priority.[11]

A major step in the development of a comprehensive health policy took place at the end of 1981 when the then Minister for Social Affairs, Pierre Marc Johnson, requested that the Council of Social Affairs examine appropriate strategies for health promotion. A task force of eighteen experts from a variety of health and related areas was established under the presidency of former deputy minister of Social Affairs, Dr Jacques Brunet. A report, entitled *Objective: Health*, was presented to the minister in August 1984. The task force took an ecological approach to the concept of health, recognizing the many physical, social, economic, and work-related factors that have an impact upon health-status outcomes. Health was defined very broadly as a process whereby an individual adapts to the environment.

According to the ecological approach, the organization of the medical-care system is only one of the issues to be addressed in the formulation of a comprehensive health policy. The task force report surveyed changes in the health status of Quebeckers and examined the main factors affecting health. It was found that there had been a significant improvement in life expectancy between 1974 and 1984. Much of this gain was the result of reduced infant-mortality rates. In 1971, Quebec had the highest rate in Canada but, by 1982, it had steadily fallen to become the lowest (Government of Quebec 1984: 28). A substantial reduction in male deaths from cardiac disease after 1976 was observed. Areas where fewer gains had been made were identified, and a number of both general and specific priority health-improvement objectives were suggested. It was recognized that, while some of the specific objectives had a medical bias, their achievement would require action extending well beyond the health-care system. In particular, the close relationship between poverty and ill health, a relationship found in studies of other countries, was singled out for attention (Government of Quebec 1984: 81–6).[12]

The findings of the task force report were presented to a variety of conferences and meetings in 1984 and 1985, including two national conferences. Within Quebec, regional health-promotion conferences were organ- ized in 1985 and 1986, at which the task force's recommendations were the subject of debate. Departments of community health have endorsed the report as an appropriate framework for use when devising more specific objectives, programs, and health targets (Pineault, Contandriopoulos, and Lessard 1985: 407). Thus, in addition to achieving a range of medical-care objectives, Quebec policy makers have made considerable progress towards the development of a policy that aims to promote the health of the population rather than merely to provide access to services for the treatment of disease.

Health Services in Australia

Developments in relation to the Australian health-care delivery system reflect the more centralized nature of the federation: the Commonwealth has played an important innovating role, and there has been more joint decision making than in Canada. The Whitlam government's proposals for reform of health insurance were only one part of the policy package formulated while the party was in opposition. Before gaining office, Mr Hayden, shadow minister for Health and Social Welfare, announced the following proposals:

1 To set up a National Hospitals and Health Services Commission to become involved cooperatively with the states to provide an adequate, planned development of rationalised health services, to develop peripheral general hospitals, and to set up community health centres.
2 To upgrade the status and role of the general practitioner by undergraduate education in community medicine, the support of expanded training for family practice, and the provision of the supporting community health staff and facilities in a system primarily coordinated by the general practitioner.
3 To introduce a system of universal health insurance.
4 To develop nursing home and domiciliary services.
5 To start a national school dental health program.
6 To undertake a national program on Aboriginal health.
7 To make preventive, occupational and rehabilitation services key elements in the health program.
8 To assist the states to integrate psychiatric inpatient services with general hospital services and to give priority to the development of community mental health services.
9 To develop systems for ongoing evaluation of the programs. (quoted in Sax 1984: 101–2)

Many of these proposals were an expansion of policies that had been developed in the states during the 1960s. In New South Wales, in particular, plans had been formulated to establish community-based services, which would replace many institutional services. Programs for the care of the aged had been implemented, and some integration of mental-health services with other parts of the health system had taken place. New South Wales had begun to establish community health centres that accommodated child-health, dental-health, and mental-health services. Health-education teams worked from these centres, some of which also provided rehabilitation services, domiciliary nursing, and home-care services (Sax 1980: 277). The aim of these developments was to overcome problems associated with the fragmentation of services, to fill gaps in the system, and to reduce levels of institutionalization (Sax 1980: 279).

While many of these proposals for reform originated in New South Wales, they had started to spread to other states. Ideas were disseminated through the Hospitals and Allied Services Advisory Council (later called the Australian Health Ministers' Advisory Council), a body of Commonwealth and state officials that had been set up to advise Health ministers. New services similar to those of New South Wales were introduced in other states (Shea 1970: 39–55; Sax 1980: 279).

It was recognized, however, that the full development of state plans could not go ahead without federal financial assistance. In 1970, Dr Brian Shea, then director general of Medical Services in South Australia, reported that 'the inescapable fact is that all State treasuries are rapidly running out of financial resources to maintain health and hospital standards at optimal levels' (1970: 41). Prior to 1972, some Commonwealth assistance had been given for the development of domiciliary nursing services and other home-care projects, such as community centres for the aged. The latter was on a dollar-for-dollar basis. However, an upper limit had been placed on the amount of Commonwealth support. State officials believed that further progress required federal-government cooperation in the form of increased funding (Shea 1970: 55).[13]

State plans to expand health services accorded with Labor's traditional policy preferences. One of the avenues through which these proposals found their way into Labor policy was through the office of the leader of the opposition, Mr Whitlam, who was keenly interested in the problems being experienced in the rapidly expanding outer areas of major cities. These suburbs were undersupplied with facilities and services in a range of areas. Staff from the Whitlam electoral office, located in an outer Sydney suburb, were in regular contact with officials in the New South Wales Department of Health and were supplied with research papers and the details of policy proposals.[14]

Soon after Labor assumed office, the decision to establish the Hospitals and Health Services Commission (HHSC) was announced. Pending the passage of the necessary legislation, an interim committee was set up under the chairmanship of Dr Sidney Sax, previously director of Geriatric Services and, later, director of Research and Planning in the New South Wales Health Department. In May 1973, this committee produced an interim report proposing a community health program for Australia. The committee envisaged 'a major Community Health Program to develop facilities and services in a coordinated manner for the provision and planning of prevention, treatment, rehabilitation and related welfare aspects of community health' (HHSC Interim Committee 1973: 28).

The committee stressed that services should be provided by teams of health professionals. As in Quebec, community centres were to have outreach programs and social-advocacy functions. The committee was of the view that there is value in a diverse and experimental range of services and did not envisage a uniform set of services. Rather, the committee recommended that 'creative use should be made of any differences in organisation or in particular lines of interest at the local, regional or State level. The deliberate promotion of individual projects, linked with evaluation studies, would enable data to be obtained on a range of developments and permit useful comparisons' (HHSC Interim Committee 1973: 9).

On the politically sensitive issue of methods of physician remuneration, the report was vague. It suggested that a variety of payment methods could be used and said that current arrangements need not necessarily be changed. However, the benefits of salaried employment such as superannuation and annual and study leave were mentioned, indicating that the committee hoped that some doctors would accept salaried posts.

The community health program was to be funded by a combination of block grants to the states and specific grants for special projects. In order that development could be coordinated to avoid the problems of fragmentation and duplication, the committee recommended that HHSC approve all grants.

There are many similarities between the Australian proposals and those of the Castonguay Commission. These include emphasis on previously neglected areas such as rehabilitation and prevention, community participation, and the geographical redistribution of services. However, whereas the Quebec reforms envisaged a reorientation of the whole health and social-welfare systems, the Australian programs were to be complementary to the hospital, and medical services funded by the health-insurance plan.

A fragmentation of responsibility at the federal level presented difficulties for the HHSC. Health functions were divided among the Department of Social Security, the Department of Health, and the HHSC. In addition, a social-welfare commission was established with the result that there was some overlap between the functions of the two commissions. This division of responsibility made coordination difficult. In addition, the government was aware that it had been elected for only three years and wanted to get its programs underway quickly (Sax 1984: 103). Even before the HHSC interim report was released, a number of special-purpose and welfare grants had been announced so that the coordinated policy development envisaged by the HHSC did not fully materialize (Sax 1984: 104–8).

Nevertheless, between 1973 and 1975, Australian health services were expanded significantly, through both joint federal–state action and federal cooperation with community groups and other non-government organizations. As in Quebec, there were divergent views about the goals of the community-health program. The more traditional view is that centres should provide both curative and preventive care. A second view eschews a 'patient' orientation and adopts a broader conception of health. In this approach, community health centres should focus on the needs of the whole community and should provide social and welfare services as well as health-education and treatment services. In practice, most Australian community health centres have tended to combine elements of both approaches (Andersen 1984: 6; Milio: 1983: 185–92).

The HHSC gave priority to programs designed to meet certain 'urgent needs' according to a set of indicators that had been developed. For example, areas of 'health scarcity' were identified, where general practitioner/population ratios were particularly low or where there was a high proportion of handicapped or multiproblem individuals or families. By 1976, it was estimated that services had been improved for about half of the 15 to 20 per cent of people who lived in underserviced areas in both metropolitan and rural locations. Services for migrants were given priority, both in terms of the obvious need for interpreter services and in terms of the different kinds of services that people from other countries were accustomed to using. Other priorities were health services for Aboriginal people, the aged, the handicapped, and alcohol- and drug-dependent people, and occupational health and health education. Thirty-seven training programs for health workers were established, including the Family Medicine Program conducted by the Royal Australian College of General Practitioners. By November 1975, 727 different projects, employing 2,200 people, were in operation. While nearly half of these programs were set up in New South Wales, only a very few health centres in that state provided medical services. This reflects the strong private-practice orientation of the New South Wales branch of the medical profession (HHSC 1976: 1–89).

The division of power between the two levels of government did not present great difficulties during the implementation process.[15] Soon after his appointment, Dr Sax visited all the states, talked with politicians and officials, and asked that consideration be given to proposals that might be put forward to the commission. Joint federal–state committees of officials were established, comprising two or three representatives of the Commonwealth and three state officials. In practice, large groups of up to twenty state representatives who were interested in various aspects of policy often attended meetings. In Dr Sax's opinion, these committees of officers functioned well.

At the political level, the only strong opposition came from the state of Victoria. As mentioned in chapter 6, both the Victorian Health minister and the secretary of the Department of Health were ideologically opposed to Labor's policies. Owing to a provision of the Victorian Hospitals and Charities Act (1958), the HHSC was able to work directly with community groups and non-government agencies, enabling many programs to be initiated. At the end of 1973, however, the Victorian government amended the legislation so that all new projects henceforth required ministerial approval. Despite these difficulties, 146 different programs had been established in Victoria by 1975.

The Queensland government was willing to accept federal funding for approved projects but insisted that conditions be reduced to a minimum. The main difference of opinion between the HHSC and the state centred upon whether community-health centres should provide medical services. Here the influence of the medical profession is again apparent. Queensland had established health centres of its own prior to 1972 that employed health professionals and social workers but not doctors. The HHSC view was that community centres located in areas where there was a shortage of doctors should provide medical services. This policy was opposed by the Queensland government, so that the central view did not prevail.

There were few political difficulties between the HHSC and the remaining four state governments. Interaction with the government of Tasmania was amicable, but the strong opposition of the Tasmanian Society of General Practitioners was an obstacle to program development. Satisfactory arrangements were negotiated with South Australia, Western Australia, and New South Wales. Overall, as Dr Sax remembers the implementation process, the main problems arose from 'personalities' and were sometimes exacerbated by party political differences.

The second main area of HHSC responsibility was to formulate a hospital-development program. There were two parts of the hospital policy. The first was a program to renovate and upgrade existing facilities, and the second was a new building program. In the non-controversial area of renovation, work proceeded smoothly, and the facilities in many institutions were improved. The hospital-building program, however, was controversial and received wide publicity.

Many of the problems in this area were related to the approach taken by the prime minister. Mr Whitlam was determined to ensure that outer urban areas would be furnished with hospital facilities and was prepared to use the Commonwealth government's constitutional power to establish Commonwealth hospitals, if necessary. He sometimes bypassed both the HHSC and the Minister for Health and undertook negotiations in relation to hospital construction directly with premiers. From a HHSC viewpoint, this approach disrupted planning, as did the haste with which many decisions were made. The 1973–4 budget, for example, provided an allocation for hospital construction, but planning and negotiations with the states were not sufficiently advanced to allow the money to be spent (Scotton 1978: 107; Sax 1984: 118–22).

The concern that some states might not agree to provide free care for Medibank patients in public hospitals appears to have influenced the prime minister's decision to press ahead with the establishment of Commonwealth hospitals. In 1974, he wrote to the premiers of three states, proposing that several federal hospitals be built. The offers were all rejected. In an agreement made directly between Mr Whitlam and the premier of Tasmania, the decision was taken to develop a large new hospital in Launceston (Sax 1984: 119). The HHSC was instructed to work with the new Department of Urban and Regional Development and the Commonwealth Department of Health to develop plans for federal hospitals. However, the HHSC took the view that 'an equitable spatial distribution of hospitals would improve the efficiency and effectiveness of services only if the facilities were part of a comprehensive, integrated system, planned and managed by a single authority' (Sax 1984: 119). Eventually, the prime minister accepted the commission's arguments, and proposals to establish Commonwealth hospitals lapsed. A hospital-development program, for which $107.2 million was allocated in the 1975–6 budget, was launched in cooperation with the states, despite resistance to federal intervention by some state governments (Scotton 1978: 107).

If Commonwealth hospitals had been established, they would have been under the control of a non-Labor government between 1975 and 1983, which might have had significant implications for the health system. Eager to reduce federal responsibility for health expenditures, the Fraser government may simply have handed these hospitals over to the states. However, control of these institutions would have been an attractive proposition for private enterprise and the medical profession, and part of the Fraser government's health policy was to strengthen the role of the private-hospital sector. By 1982 this policy had given rise to what critics called the beginning of a 'medical-industrial complex.' In about one-third of Victorian for-profit hospitals, doctors or their relatives were either directors or shareholders and, after only three years of operation, a subsidiary of an American company had taken control of 6 per cent of Australian acute-care private hospitals (Morley, Taylor, and Opit 1982: 25–9). The sale of Commonwealth hospitals would thus have suited the ideological position and the budgetary objectives of the Fraser government and, moreover, would have met some of the aims of hospital-based medical specialists. One of the limiting factors in the New South Wales doctors' strike in 1984–5 was that there were insufficient acute-care private hospitals in which resigning specialists could practise. New South Wales has a smaller proportion of private hospital beds than any other state (Chesterman 1986: 80). A larger private-hospital sector would have served to strengthen the bargaining position of the medical profession and would almost certainly have jeopardized the success of future Labor initiatives.

Under the Fraser government, federal financial support for both hospital construction and the community-health program was gradually withdrawn. Federal funding under the hospital-development program was reduced from $108 million in 1976–7 to $50 million in 1977–8. The Commonwealth announced at the 1978 Premiers' Conference that assistance under the hospital program would cease, except for a commitment to meet 50 per cent of the cost of the first stage of the Launceston hospital development. Funding under the community-health program fell from $79.1 million in 1977–8 to $52.6 million in constant dollars in 1978–9. The community-health grant and the grant for the school dental service were absorbed into the general tax-sharing allocation (Ferber 1980: 351–7; Sax 1984: 140–3). In June 1978, the Minister for Health announced that HHSC had in many ways achieved its purpose, and in August the commission was abolished (Ferber 1980: 357).

The Labor government that came to power in 1983 was committed to the reintroduction of universal health insurance but had virtually no policies in relation to health services. Federal grants under the community-health program were restored to the levels of 1975–6, although no adjustment was made for the interim increase in population. Thus the states were able to establish some new projects, but the federal government has chosen not to take an active policy role and has placed very few conditions on the grant. This position is partly a reflection of the unfavourable economic and ideological climate that has led to priority being placed on financial and economic policy and partly a reflection of the fact that the Hawke government is less activist in its approach to health and other social policies than previous federal Labor governments.

There has, however, been a modest effort to expand community-based services, particularly for children and the aged. A new Commonwealth department of community services was established in 1984. It took responsibility for the child-care, rehabilitation, and residential programs previously run by the Department of Social Security, and for nursing homes, which were previously a Health Department function. Thus, community-based health and social services were combined in one portfolio. The department provides services in cooperation with states, local government, and non-government organizations.

Since 1984, existing programs have been steadily expanded and new programs have been introduced. Funding for child care has been increased substantially. A new family-support program began in January 1987. Rehabilitation services and services for the homeless have been expanded, and attention has been given to the provision of services in previously undersupplied outer urban and rural areas.[16]

In 1985, the Home and Community Care (HACC) program was introduced on the basis of recommendations made in several reports and inquiries undertaken during the previous ten years. The details of policy were worked out in cooperation with the states, service providers, and non-government organizations. Program objectives are to promote the development of a comprehensive range of home-care and community services for the aged and disabled. Four existing conditional grants for home care were grouped together into a single, federal–state cost-shared program. Agreements have been made with all states under the conditions of which decisions relating to the establishment of new services and changes in resource allocation are to be made jointly. The states are free to decide whether to provide services directly or whether to provide assistance to local government and other agencies. During the period of the agreements, which is initially three years, the Commonwealth financial contribution is to increase annually by 20 per cent in money terms (Gray 1990).

The policies of the Department of Community Services[17] have been uncontroversial and represent a successful exercise in joint implementation. Although there have been funding increases of up to several hundred per cent for some programs under the Hawke government, the federal contribution was very low under the Fraser non-Labor government, and total outlays are still small. However, if this steady, incremental development were to be sustained over a period of time, a significant expansion of community services would result.

Another innovation that may have an impact on Australian health policy in the future was the appointment of the Better Health Commission in March 1985. Announcing the decision, the federal Health minister said that 'the Better Health Commission represents the first concerted national effort to change the basic direction of health policy in this country. For far too long, the emphasis on health care in Australia has been on illness treatment rather than prevention ... What we need to develop is a national preventive health strategy to support the already extensive work in the curative and research fields.'[18] The Commission's three-volume report was released in November 1986 and contains extensive information on the health status of Australians, on the incidence of preventable disease, and on the health problems of groups at additional risk. After deliberation, the commission selected three areas in which it recommended that the development of health goals and strategies should be given priority: cardiovascular disease, nutrition, and injury. Other areas it decided warranted urgent attention are cancer, communicable diseases, and mental health. Extensive recommendations were made with the intention of establishing a framework for a national commitment to preventive health and health promotion, including the appointment of 'a high level national body ... to provide leadership ... and to act as a focus for health promotion and the prevention of ill-health.' Budgetary concerns have been given priority over service provision by the Hawke government, but if new money were to be made available for health, the information presented by the commission would provide a valuable guide for policy makers.[19]

Conclusion

Both the Australian and Canadian federal systems have allowed reforms of the health-care delivery system to be implemented in response to criticisms of policies that concentrated on providing access only to curative medical services. In Canada, where the provinces have primary responsibility for health policy, Quebec has undertaken a radical reform of its whole health-care system. During the same period, other provinces have pursued ad hoc policies designed to de-emphasize curative medical services with the object of achieving containment of health-care costs. The fact that policy making in Quebec has differed so radically from that in other provinces is not attributable to constitutional or even to financial constraints, but rather is explained by political factors. Quebec has been as successful as other provinces in achieving control of health expenditures (Barer and Evans 1989) and has demonstrated that the provision of an alternative range of services is possible, even within the context of budgetary restraint. The policy response in Quebec, as in Saskatchewan in the 1940s and 1950s, reflects the strong public demand for reform and the subsequent election of successive governments committed to the implementation of a wide range of social-welfare innovations.

Australian policy development, by contrast, took place through joint federal-state action. In a process that strongly resembles the introduction of national health insurance in Canada, policies for the expansion of community-based services were developed in the states and were later taken up by a federal Labor government, which was committed to extensive innovation in social policy. As in Quebec, the early 1970s provided political opportunities for innovation. After twenty-three years of non-Labor federal government, there were widespread demands for reform, a situation reflected in Labor's 1972 campaign slogan 'It's Time for Change.'

Health-services development was possible in both federations when political conditions were favourable. The process through which reforms were implemented is different and reflects the different degrees of centralization in the two federations. These factors serve to demonstrate that policy innovation in federations can take a variety of forms. Whether social-democratic policies are more likely to be advanced in a centralized or a decentralized federation cannot be established from this comparison of the two systems. All that can be said with certainty is that a Canadian federal government committed to health-policy reform will be constrained by its lack of constitutional and political power in the degree to which it can influence provincial policy while Australian state governments will be similarly constrained by their limited financial independence and their relative acceptance of federal domination but, as Trudeau argued, the sum of government power is not necessarily thereby diminished.

Developments in Quebec, in Australia, and in many other countries in the 1970s show that ideas are a crucial factor in an explanation of policy innovations, whatever the system of government. Countries in which policy making focused upon the development of primary care and preventive services include Britain, Germany, Sweden, France, Israel, and Yugoslavia (Blanpain 1978; Andersen 1984). The evidence suggests that the extent to which governments are likely to respond to new ideas is heavily dependent upon political, economic, and ideological factors, and that institutional factors are of relatively minor significance. The Fraser and Hawke governments in Australia had the same opportunities to promote the expansion of health services as did the Whitlam government but chose to gradually withdraw from the policy area in the one case and to maintain the status quo in the other. The Canadian provinces are all in the same institutional position as the province of Quebec. Their inaction is partly explained by an absence of strong public pressure for reform, by concern about rapidly rising costs, and by the constraints imposed by economic recession. Two other important factors distinguish the circumstances in Quebec from those in the other provinces. First, the Quebec reforms began before the onset of recession. Changes in the timing of the innovations may have produced a different outcome. Second, the problem of extra-billing was resolved in Quebec in 1970, whereas most other provinces had still to face a confrontation with the medical profession on this issue. The tense political circumstances surrounding extra-billing and control of provincial fee schedules were not conducive to introducing other policies opposed by the medical profession.

8

Federalism and the Determinants of Health Policy

Health-policy developments in Canada and Australia have been examined in the preceding chapters on a case-by-case basis. In this final chapter, the evidence as a whole is surveyed in an attempt to arrive at some general conclusions about the main determinants of policy and the role of federal institutions in policy processes.

Clearly the role played by the medical profession was crucial in both countries. But doctors will not be able to gain all of their objectives. The circumstances in which they failed to do so will be examined below. Political parties, party competition, and elections were central factors in policy development. Ideas, disseminated between the jurisdictions of the two federations and internationally, were an important force. Ideological conflict surrounded policy innovation in both countries, but has been far more intense and enduring in Australia. The importance of the role played by the bureaucracy varied according to circumstances. When the medical profession opposed new developments, as was most often the case, the main principles and outlines of policy were fought out publicly in the political arena. A much more closed decision-making process took place when doctors and governments were in general agreement. At these times, the role of civil servants was more important.

All of these policy influences operated together in institutional settings of divided power. It is clearly very difficult to isolate the independent effect of federal institutions from this array of forces. However, it is equally difficult to find concrete evidence in the case-studies to support the main contentions of the 'orthodox' federal theories discussed in chapter 1. In the mid-1980s, the Canadian and Australian health systems were remarkably similar. Yet these outcomes were achieved through quite different federal processes. At the very least, Canadian experience demonstrates that social-democractic programs can be implemented in a highly decentralized political system and that national standards can be developed and preserved. Health policy remains primarily a provincial responsibility, but the federal government has played a crucial role in development. In contrast, public health insurance has not been established as a permanent component of the Australian health system, despite the high level of centralization in the post-war period. Non-Labor sections of the medical profession remain opposed to Medicare, and it seems highly likely that the system will be at least partly reprivatized when Labor loses office at the Commonwealth level. Taken together, then, Canadian and Australian policy patterns show that centralization is neither a necessary nor a sufficient condition for the achievement of social-democatic reforms. Overall, the evidence from the studies provides little support for traditional theories.

In contrast, the evidence from health suggests that the 'revisionist' theory is a more useful guide to the operation of federal systems. Canadian and early Australian experience shows that divided power can give rise to the coexistence of a number of activist governments, particularly when that power is highly decentralized. According to this view, federalism may operate as an expansionary rather than a contradictory force on the growth of government activity. However, as with 'orthodox' theories, we should be careful not to attribute too much explanatory power to the institutional variable. First, the 'revisionist' theory is a very poor guide to the politics of Australian federalism in the post-war period. Second, decentralization does not necessarily give rise to the emergence of activist governments: some provinces and some states were relatively inactive during most of the period under review. Third, centralization and decentralization can have quite different effects on the social-democratic programs, depending on the other forces at work at a given moment. For example, central responsibility for national standards provided the Trudeau government with a dream opportunity to initiate a popular policy (the preservation of univeral health insurance) while leaving the provinces with the invidious task of negotiating a settlement with the medical profession. In Australia, however, centralization has been one of the reasons that non-Labor federal governments have been able to terminate Labor innovations in the post-war period almost at will.

The Determinants of Health Policy

We turn now to an examination of the social, political, and economic forces that have been channelled through federal institutions in the process of developing health policy. The discussion below is arranged in four sections. In the first, the major policy deteminants are identified. In the second part, orthodox federal theory is assessed in relation to the case-study evidence. The extent to which a 'revisionist' approach is useful explanatory tool is the subject of the third section. Finally, the possibility of building a universally valid theory of federalism is considered.

Political Parties, Party Competition, and Elections

The impact of political parties, party competition, and elections was of central importance in the processes of policy making. In terms of putting health on the political agenda, in formulating the principles if not the details of policy proposals, and in generating the necessary commitment to embark upon politically difficult courses of action, political parties played a major role in both federations. Elections were important in bringing to power parties that were committed to reform. At other times, the prospect of an election moved a reluctant government to action. Party competition operated differently in the two countries, however. In Canada, a high level of consensus on most aspects of policy developed after initial disagreement, whereas in Australia the two major parties have vehemently and enduringly opposed each other's health schemes. The comparatively steady, incremental nature of Canadian policy development appears to be attributable largely to the high level of party agreement. In contrast, the competing ideological perspectives of Australia's major parties are the principal reasons for the frequent and major changes in policy direction.

The emergence and electoral success of the social democratic CCF in western Canada put health insurance on the political agenda, particularly in Saskatchewan and British Columbia. A Liberal government came to power in 1933 in British Columbia with the promise to introduce public health insurance. At the election, the first contested by the CCF, the new party polled 31.1 per cent of the vote. After years of delay, the Liberal government of Saskatchewan passed health-insurance legislation just before the 1944 election, in which it was heavily defeated. The growing electoral strength of the CCF and the reform policies developed by the Progressive Conservatives in opposition forced a reluctant Mackenzie King government to address social-policy issues during the Second World War. A major factor in the St Laurent government's decision to proceed with hospital insurance in 1957 was the forthcoming federal election. The 1960 Saskatchewan election campaign, in which the Liberal opposition supported the medical profession, was virtually transformed into a referendum on Medicare. At the same time, the federal Liberal party, which had reformulated its policies while in opposition, was pressing the Diefenbaker government to take action on national medicare insurance. When in government, the Liberal party kept that commitment despite opposition from some members of Cabinet, some provincial governments, and most doctors. Finally, electoral politics was a major motivating force behind the passage of the 1984 Canada Health Act.

Thus, although scholars generally agree that there is a high level of ideological convergence between Canada's two main political parties (McLeod 1982; Fox 1982), different positions have been taken on the controversial aspects of health policy. Decisions to support or oppose various policies were heavily influenced by electoral considerations. After initial disagreement, however, both major parties were prepared to support policy innovations. Federal hospital-insurance legislation was passed unanimously by the House of Commons and the Senate in 1957, Medicare legislation passed by a vote of 172 to 2, and the Canada Health Act was endorsed unanimously in 1984.

In the process of putting health on the political agenda and campaigning for reform, the part played by the CCF-NDP was crucial. Apart from its role in government and opposition in the western provinces and in Ontario, the party had a strong influence on federal politics. Members have persistently kept social-policy issues on the agenda both inside and outside the House of Commons. In the opinion of former minister for National Health and Welfare, Monique Bégin, both major parties have been concerned to prevent the NDP from increasing its share of the vote, which has consistently hovered around 18 per cent. In the process, both parties have 'systematically remained centrist' and have 'regularly stolen NDP policies and ideas.'[1] Mme Bégin's view of the role of party competition is supported by McLeod (1982: 315), who argues that 'third parties like the [CCF-NDP], and the Ginger group before it, have served to popularize radical policy innovations and to push the government party off its conservative stance in the political dead-centre. The influence of third parties on policy has far exceeded their power as measured in number of seats won. The origins of such positive departures from the middle of the road as old age pensions, unemployment insurance, hospitalization insurance and medicare can be attributed largely to third parties.'

In contrast with Canada, Australia has not had an electorally successful third party on the left of the political spectrum. The Country-cum-

National party has taken a position seldom distinguishable from that of the Liberal party on social-policy issues. The Democratic Labor party, which split from Labor in 1955, was primarily concerned with anti-communism, moral conservatism, defence, and keeping Labor out of office. More recent third parties, the Australia party and the Australian Democrats, were established to occupy a central position between the major parties. Party competition has thus been primarily between Labor and non-Labor.

In the first half of the century it was customary to explain Australian politics in terms of the 'initiative-resistance' thesis.[2] Labor, the working-class party, was seen as the party of initiative, promoting policies financed from taxation. Non-Labor, representing the owners of capital and financial interests, was the party of negativism and resistance, strongly opposed to policies requiring increased taxation. This thesis has become increasingly discredited since the 1950s. Analysts have argued that the only differences between the policies of the two sides of politics are differences of emphasis (Davies 1964: 124–6). Aitkin (1977: 1–2) explains the perceived convergence in terms of the parties' needs to gain the support of the middle ground of the electorate. Australian governments, he argues, 'have been reluctant to undo the work of their predecessors, whatever noises they may have made before and during election campaigns. The relatively even division of the Australian electorate at any time, the ever-present possibility that the next election will see the replacement of the party in power by its rival have fostered on both sides of politics, a cautious, incremental approach to government.'

While this argument may be valid in some policy fields, it certainly does not hold in health where the initiative-resistance thesis retains a high level of plausibility. Early in the century the labour movement promoted the idea of publicly provided, tax-financed hospital, medical, and public-health services. Labor governments in New South Wales, Queensland, and, after 1935, Tasmania extended the range of available services and increased access to them. The difference between the parties at the federal level is illustrated by the policies advanced in the pre- and post-war years. Non-Labor promoted a limited system of compulsory, contributory insurance in 1938 and introduced voluntary health insurance in the early 1950s. In contrast, Labor attempted to implement a comprehensive, tax-financed national health service in the 1940s. Party policies have been based on the different principles underpinning these schemes ever since. Labor has sought to provide universal access to services and has been willing to assume responsibility for a major proportion of health expenditures and for increased levels of direct service provision. Non-Labor, in contrast, has sought to keep government intervention in the private medical market to a minimum. It has been unwilling to assume responsibility for the organization and provision of services and has attempted to limit public-sector financial commitments by fostering private rather than public insurance. Party policies clearly favour different constituencies: Labor's policies are of most benefit to low-income earners whereas private health insurance with tax-deductible premiums favours higher-income earners and the medical profession.

Health was a major issue during the 1969, 1972, 1974, and 1983 federal elections and emerged again as a contested issue in the election held in July 1987. The Liberal party announced its intention, if returned to powers, to reprivatize insurance arrangements. Tax concessions were to be offered to encourage twelve million people to opt out of the public insurance system and to take out private health insurance. Medicare coverage was to be retained only for pensioners and other low-income groups. Former Liberal party spokesperson for health, James Porter, estimated that the expenditure savings to the Commonweatlh would be in the order of $3000 million per annum (*Age* 13 April: 1, 3). In response to strong criticism, however, these proposals were modified during the election campaign, but, as Labor was returned to office, national health insurance was maintained, at least for another three years.

The Australian situation therefore contrasts markedly with that in Canada, where there was all-party support at the federal level for the 1984 Canada Health Act that preserved and strengthened the public health-insurance system. The Conservative government enforced the provisions of the act after its election in 1984 with the result that there is far greater policy continuity in Canada than in Australia. These contrasting patterns of party competition are related to different degrees of polarization in the two political communities and, in this, ideology is an important factor.

The Role of Ideology

Tuohy (1989b) argues persuasively that ideology is a central element in an explanation of differing public-policy outcomes in Canada and the United States, countries that she points out are otherwise more striking in their similarities than in their differences. Although an essentially similar medical technology has evolved in the two countries, government intervention in health is much greater in Canada (Tuohy 1989b: 402–4). Following Horowitz's (1966) adaptation of the Hartz theory of the founding of new societies,[3] her explanation is that the ideological spectrum in

Canada is more fully developed than that of its neighbour. The spectrum in the United States is

occupied almost entirely by liberal pluralism, ranging from a thorough-going defense of individualism (as has often been noted, what American 'conservatives' have to preserve is eighteenth and nineteenth century liberalism) through 'interest group' liberalism (emphasising the countervailing power of groups representing a variety of interests) to 'neo-mercantile' and 'welfare state' liberalism (emphasising, to varying degrees, the necessity for cooperation between private groups and the state to minimise destructive competition and the responsibility of the state to provide a 'safety net' for the victims of the competition market). (Tuohy 1989b: 389)

In contrast, a 'complete' ideological spectrum, according to Horowitz (1966: 143–4), is more extensive. It ranges from feudalism or Toryism on the right 'through liberal whig to liberal democrat to socialist' on the left. Feudal or Tory values include the concept of 'the organic, corporate, hierarchical community.' Unlike liberalism, Toryism is not averse to concentrations of state power. In an organic, hierarchical community those holding privileged positions are thought to have a responsibility to support redistributive policies (Tuohy 1989b: 395–6).

Tuohy argues that the Canadian ideological spectrum, like that of the United States, is dominated by liberal pluralism but differs in that it encompasses two additional elements: Toryism on the right and socialism on the left. According to Hartz, British North America is a liberal fragment but, where Toryism was renounced by American liberals at the time of the war of independence, a Tory 'streak' or 'touch' was retained and preserved by Canadians, enabling socialist ideas to take root in Canada because they could be accommodated in an ideological climate that already incorporated non-liberal elements (Horowitz 1966: 150–9). As a result, Canada has developed a distinctive political culture, which includes 'tory-touched' liberals less distrustful of concentrated power than their United States counterparts; 'red tories' supportive of redistributive policies ...; democratic socialists willing to pursue collectivist goals through the institutions of the liberal state' (Tuohy 1989b: 398). Thus there is both more support for and less distrust of government-sponsored policies of redistribution in Canada than in the United States.

Tuohy's analysis is supported by the conclusions of King's (1973) study of the scope of government activity in Britain, France, Germany, Canada, and the United States. King found that different attitudes towards the appropriate role of the state are of crucial importance in explaining why the public sector is smaller in the United States than in the other four countries. Social democrats, committed to making extensive use of the state, are an important political force in Canada and Europe but not in the United States. But it is equally important, King argues, that 'conservatives in the other four countries ... are also not consistently anti-statist in attitude; on the contrary they often express a highly exalted view of the role of the state in economic and social life' (1973: 419).

According to Donald Smiley, Toryism is an important force in Canadian politics. It is manifest in the high priority placed upon order and stability and in a national distaste for conflict and unpredictable change.[4] The relative lack of opposition to a large role for the state and the preference for consensus and orderly change are consistent with the steady incremental development and preservation of public health insurance.

If the Canadian ideological spectrum, as developed by Horowitz and Tuohy, is compared with that of Australia, there appears to be considerable similarity on the left and in the centre, but not on the right. The strength of social-democratic ideas is evidence of a radical egalitarianism in Australia in 'the spirit of the Chartists and of Cobbett' (Hartz 1964: 4).[5] Hartz was in error when he proclaimed the 'nationalization' of the radical ethos, as historians such as McCarty (1973), Bolton (1973), and Hirst (1984) have pointed out, for Australia, like the United States and Canada, is also dominated by liberal pluralism. However, there is a radical strand in Australia, and the Labor party, like the CCF-NDP, has vigorously promoted the use of state power to implement social-democratic policies. The centre of the ideological spectrum, too, appears to be similar, occupied by those of roughly 'liberal interventionist' persuasion. But, on the right, there are strong contrasts. Australian political culture appears to be without the moderating influence of Toryism. As in the United States, there is no politically significant group that can be equated with those Canadians identify as Red Tories. There have been individuals, such as Sir Thomas Playford, non-Labor premier of South Australia from 1938 to 1965, who supported an extensive state role in both economic and social policy. However, few on the non-Labor side of politics have supported more than a slow expansion of benefits under existing programs, and social-policy issues have often been contested in highly ideological and adversarial language. The oscillation between systems of public and private health insurance reflects a high level of polarization in the community on the appropriate social-policy role of the state. The adversarial nature of party competition and radical changes in policy direction are accepted, and there is less opposition to privatization. It is difficult to imagine a non-Labor leader declaring, as Brian Mulroney has done, that 'universal programs are a sacred trust.' Indeed, since the introduction of means-testing for family allowances by the Labor government in 1986, a policy change that did not result in political costs for the government, despite the opposition of the women's movement, Medicare is Australia's only remaining universal program, and its continuation again appears to be coming under threat.[6]

In ideological terms, then, health-policy experience can be used to support an argument that Australian political culture stands somewhere between that of Canada and of the United States. In the United States, where the ideological spectrum is said to consist almost entirely of liberal pluralism, government responsibility is limited to providing access to care for the aged and the very poor. The distribution of services for other groups is a function of the market, a policy very similar to that proposed by the Australian Liberal party at the 1987 election. The promotion of state responsibility in Canada and Australia can be seen as reflecting ideological spectrums that extend farther to the left than that of the United States. Opposition to government intervention in Australia and the United States might denote a right that does not extend to Red Toryism. Alternatively, to avoid the pitfalls of the Hartz and Horowitz theses, it could be argued simply that, while all three countries are dominated by liberalism, 'new' or welfare-state liberalism is strong in Canada and Australia but weak in the United States, whereas liberal individualism, strong in the United States and Australia, is weak in Canada. Such an argument, however, misses the positive view of the role of the state that King and others have found among Canadian conservatives and that appears to have played an important role in the development of the Canadian welfare state.

The Influence of the Bureaucracy

In general terms, the evidence from health policy is in accordance with Heclo's findings from Sweden and Britain that civil servants played an important part 'in giving concrete substance to new policy initiatives and in elaborating already established approaches' (1974: 304). However, it would be a mistake to attribute primacy to the role of the bureaucracy in health policy. First, policies were frequently formulated by parties or party executives during periods of opposition. The Political Labor League of

New South Wales developed detailed policy proposals that the party attempted to implement when it gained power in 1910. The Queensland Labor party, the Saskatchewan CCF, the Canadian federal Liberal party, the Quebec Liberal party, the Australian Labor party, and the Ontario Liberal party – all developed reform proposals while out of office. In the 1950s, the Australian non-Labor government implemented policy that had been formulated by the AMA. In some cases these policies were general and required further elaboration; in others, such as the Australian Labor party's Medibank and Medicare proposals and the Quebec reforms, detailed study and planning had been undertaken before the sponsoring party came to power.

A second factor, which had the effect of reducing the importance of the bureaucratic role, is the use of outside policy advisers. The Saskatchewan government in the 1940s, the Quebec government of the early 1970s, and the Australian Whitlam and Hawke governments – all drew experts from outside the permanent civil service to assist with policy implementation. Third, and most obviously, the options open to officials, like those open to ministers and other policy actors, were heavily circumscribed by the need to develop proposals that had some prospect of acceptance by the medical profession. To take just one example, the medical-care insurance system introduced in Saskatchewan in 1962 bore no resemblance to the locally controlled medical-care system based on the existing municipal doctor scheme, which had been proposed originally by the Health Services Planning Commission. Under the commission's scheme, a comprehensive set of services was to be developed at the municipal level. Doctors were to be paid by a mixture of salary, capitation, and fees as appropriate. When Medicare was finally introduced, it simply underwrote existing patterns of private medical practice. Moreover, the government was forced to concede all parts of its policy concerning the method of remibursing doctor's fees.

On some occasions, the bureaucracy played a central role in policy development. Such was the case in both Canada and Australia at the federal level during the Second World War, when national proposals were being formulated, and again in Canada during the 1970s, when cost-control became a dominant issue. Civil servants, especially those from Finance departments, played a key role in the move from cost-sharing to block funding. The various policies introduced by the Fraser government during the Medibank-termination process were developed at the bureaucratic level largely by officers from the coordinating departments of Treasury and Finance, and prime minister and Cabinet. However, the proposals were in line with the government's broad objectives of reducing Commonwealth expenditure and maintaining a strong sector of private hospital and medical insurance, and private medical practice. They were also in accordance with the preferred policies of the AMA. The voluntary health-insurance system reintroduced in 1981 was well known so that decisions had to be made only about the details of the scheme.

Thus, the importance of civil servants in policy development has fluctuated. In general, the main contours and principles of new policies have been fought out in the political arena, a process in which many actors and influences played important roles.

The Influence of Interest Groups

It is unnecessary to re-examine the many, varied, and frequently decisive ways in which the medical profession contributed to the shape of Canadian and Australian health policy. It is sufficient to note that doctors in both countries used internationally known arguments and strategies in their quest to maintain a high level of economic and clinical freedom. As Blanpain (1978: 217) observes, 'there is a remarkable universality in the way ... mechanisms designed to ensure professional autonomy and medical dominance of the national health program have been employed by the medical profession throughout the world.' Blanpain attributes this common approach partly to a high level of 'cross-fertilization on positions and tactics' among doctors in different countries, a process that resembles the spread of ideas in other areas of health policy (1978: 211).

In the 1970s and 1980s, Australian and Canadian doctors were less successful than formerly in achieving their goals. Significantly, the medical profession lost battles in both countries during this period on what Eckstein (1960: 89) termed 'that touchiest of all areas of policy: remuneration.' On the basis of evidence from ten countries, especially that from Britain, Sweden, and the United States, Marmor and Thomas argued in 1972 that governments could not win disputes with the profession on remuneration. Such was the case whether the issue was unit of payment (capitation, fee-for-service, salary), source of payment (patient, intermediary, government), or the system of differentiating among groups of doctors for remuneration purposes. 'Doctors,' they argued, 'get their way on methods of pay' (Marmor and Thomas 1972: 438).

Marmor and Thomas criticized Eckstein's (1960) study of the British Medical Association on a number of grounds, including his conclusion that one of the main reasons for the association's success was that negotiations with government were closed and private. The comparative evidence, Marmor and Thomas argued, showed that the medical profession was invariably successful in pay disputes, whatever the political and institutional arrangements of the country in question. They attributed this success to the 'overwhelming political resources' of physicians 'as producers of crucial service in industrial countries' and predicted that doctors would continue to succeed because 'Western industrial states will never risk a medical strike because of the high political costs associated with the interruption of personal health services, irrespective of government views on the merits of physician demands' (1972: 437).

While it is probably true that most governments would wish to avoid doctors' strikes 'at almost any cost,' the evidence from Canada and Australia suggests that governments have been rather more willing to take this risk in recent years. In addition to the more serious strikes described in earlier chapters, Canadian provincial governments have weathered a number of episodes of service disruption or 'study days' as medical associations responded to the hard line taken on medical-fee increases. However, in a significant number of cases in the 1970s and 1980s, doctors were unable to gain their objectives in pay disputes as defined by Marmor and Thomas. Quebec doctors lost the right to be paid by patients in 1970, and the struggle to retain this right was lost throughout Canada between 1984 and 1987. Australian doctors failed to gain their preferred unit of payment (fee-for-service) and preferred source of payment (patient) for work in public hospitals in 1975 and again in 1984–5.

Governments have thus achieved their policy objectives on an unprecedented number of occasions in the last two decades in both Canada and Australia. On most occasions, the issues in dispute were highly controversial and the subject of extensive public debate. The evidence would thus seem to support Eckstein's argument that the power of the medical profession is greatest when negotiations with government are closed and private. However, this is not, as Eckstein suggests, because of the nature of the negotiation process itself: as Marmor and Thomas have pointed out, the will of the medical profession has prevailed despite variations in the structure of bargaining processes between countries. Rather, private negotiations suggest that the matter under discussion is not a highly political issue. It may be that governments and the profession are in fundamental agreement on principles (Australia 1950–67) or that governments wish to avoid a public confrontation with the profession (Australia 1970–2, 1979–81). As Klein (1977: 169) argues, 'the strongest power of any interest group is implicit power: a position so strong that no open threats are needed – a recognition of indispensability which makes industrial action unnecessary.' Most important, private negotiations suggest the absence of strong public pressure for action to which the medical profession is opposed. In this situation, governments do not need to consider the demands of other groups, and neither side needs to justify its position in the public arena.

The evidence from Canadian and Australian experience shows that negotiations with doctors are likely to be open and highly controversial, either when there are strong public demands for policy changes or when governments are strongly committed to achieving their objectives despite medical opposition. In these cases, the countervailing power exerted by government and/or other groups prevented doctors from winning remuneration disputes. This finding is not inconsistent with British experience because, although Eckstein emphasized the importance of the structure of bargaining processes, he also acknowledged that the BMA case showed that 'British pressure groups are relatively weak in defense against policies for which there is strong public support' (Eckstein 1960: 106).

Strong public demands and the mobilization of groups in support of these demands are the key to understanding the reasons that Canadian doctors lost pay disputes. Large powerful unions campaigned against the Quebec specialists in 1970. The Canadian labour movement, the national and provincial health coalition groups, the Canadian Public Health Association, associations of Canadian nurses, and other 'defend Medicare' groups – all actively pressured governments to legislate to eliminate extra-billing from 1979 onwards. In Alford's (1975) terms, this political situation can be seen as the mobilization of 'repressed' interests in opposition to 'dominant' interests or 'professional monopolists.' Alford categorized the medical profession and the medical research establishment as the dominant interests in the health area because their power and resource are 'safely embedded in law, custom, professional legitimacy and the practices of many public and private organizations' (1975: 191). These groups, he argued, need not be active or cohesively organized to defend their interests. Repressed interests, however, are those groups that would benefit from equal access to health care but whose interests are not served because the necessary social institutions and political mechanisms are not in place in the organizational structure (Alford 1975: 15). The nature of institutional arrangements in America guarantees that the interests of these groups will not be met, Alford argues, unless 'extraordinary political energies' can be mobilized.

Non-medical group mobilization did emerge in Canada. Modifying

Alford's categories to fit the Canadian context, Weller (1980: 413) observed that 'challenging and repressed interests' had become 'far more aggressive' and that these groups were 'employing a wider range of tactics' than had previously been the case. Pressure from these groups, which were supported by the NDP and some provincial branches of the Liberal party, was sustained throughout the early 1980s. A reluctant federal Cabinet was eventually moved to pass the Canada Health Act in the hope of gaining political mileage for the 1984 election. Strong public support for Medicare and the mobilization of previously inactive groups can therefore be seen as the main reasons that Canadian doctors were unable to defend their economic autonomy.

There has been no comparable group mobilization in Australia (Gray 1987b). To understand the pattern of Australian health policy and the fluctuating success of the medical profession it is necessary to look more closely at public opinion.

Public Opinion

Supporters of Labor government health policies have never constituted more than a small majority of Australians in the post-war period. In contrast, as Mr Justice Hall argued in 1980, 'the nationwide demand for Medicare is an accepted fact' in Canada (p. 2). Similarly, the Task Force on the Allocation of Health Care Resources (n.d. xii), which was funded by the CMA, reported in 1983 that, 'in the course of our travels, we have found that almost all Canadians are in favour of our universal publicly funded health care system.' In the same year, an opinion poll showed that 85 per cent of Canadians supported Medicare and rated it one of the most important government programs (*Calgary Herald* 12 September 1983: A1). Even after an active campaign by the medical profession to enlist public support for its cause, 83 per cent of people opposed physician extra-billing in 1984 (*Toronto Star* 10 March 1984: A3).

Support for national health insurance is much weaker in Australia. Table 4 shows the results of selected opinions polls since 1943.

The first point of note is the significant decline in support of Labor's proposals between 1943 and 1949, a factor that may partly account for the government's inability to gain the cooperation of the medical profession. The second point is the remarkable stability of support and opposition between 1949 and 1984. A small majority of people has always supported Labor proposals, and a consistent 35 per cent or more of the population has opposed them. The third point shown in the table is the

TABLE 4
Support for Labor health policies

	1943	1947	1949	1970	1975	1984
Australia						
Support	76	66	58	54	53	57
Oppose	19	26	35	38	41	39
Undecided	5	8	7	8	1	4
Labor Voters						
Support		78	78	67	75	76
Oppose		14	16	26	19	21
Undecided		8	6	7	6	3
Liberal Voters						
Support		51	36	43	28	30
Oppose		42	57	49	65	67
Undecided		7	7	8	7	3

SOURCES: Australian Gallup Polls (Nos. 153–61, October 1943; Nos. 569–78, March 1949; Nos. 2159–74, January-March 1970); (Age Poll *Age* 12 May 1975: 5); Australian Public Opinion Polls (Poll No. 04/4/84, April 1984)
NOTE: The wording of the questions asked varied according to the policy being considered. However, the polls have been selected carefully. In each case, the question asked, in essence, whether people supported or opposed the health scheme being promoted by Labor.

polarization of opinion along party lines. Only in 1970, when dissatisfaction with the voluntary health-insurance system was widespread, were a large minority of non-Labor voters prepared to support public health insurance.

The pattern of Australian health policy can be seen, therefore, partly as a response by the major parties to the preferences of their own constituencies. Of course, as V.O. Key (1961: 456) argued, opinion does not emerge fully formed from the enviroment but is at least partly generated by the activities of political élites. However, irrespective of whether the main flow of influence is from above or below or the other way around, a very stable division of opinion has prevailed. Public health insurance does not have the strong majority support that it has in Canada.

By contrast, non-Labor governments have successfully implemented policies for which there was little public support, even among Liberal and National/Country party voters (Gray 1984: 12–13). However, non-Labor has not had to survive the political costs of active campaigns of opposition by the medical profession. Moreover, doctors enjoy high status in Australia, and studies have shown that public opinion is likely to be influenced by the prestige of those promoting an issue (Klein 1974: 414). Thus there appears to be a 'balance' among the forces in Australian health politics: non-Labor, in coalition with powerful provider interests backed by a minority of voters, and Labor, with the support of trade unions and the majority support of the unorganized, have both implemented radical policy changes.

Unlike the case in Canada, activist groups have not proliferated in the health field. The main organizations that have been involved are the Australian Council of Trade Unions, the Australian Council of Social Services, and the small Doctors' Reform Society, on the one hand, and the medical profession, private hospitals, and the voluntary health insurance funds, on the other. These groups have been unable to prevent the implementation of policies to which they were opposed in recent years. There has been no significant mobilization of non-medical health professionals or 'repressed' groups such as patients' rights associations in defence of public health insurance, although there are indications that changes may be taking place. The women's health movement is steadily gaining strength, and nurses' associations have recently become militant in support of better wages and conditions. The establishment of a network of community health centres has given rise to state and national community health associations, and a health issues centre was formed in Victoria in 1984. The centre strongly supports Medicare, the women's health movement, and locally based primary health care and prevention. However, the groups that have so far emerged seem unlikely to disturb the configuration of forces that has given Australian health policy its distinctive pattern.

In summary, there have been two sets of circumstances in which the medical profession has not been able to prevail in disputes with governments. The first is when mobilized groups and public opinion are strongly opposed to the preferred policies of the profession. The second is when committed governments are prepared to risk a withdrawal of services in the interests of achieving their policy objectives.

Up to this point we have examined the main domestic forces that have shaped health-policy development. However, as a recent and growing body of literature suggests, international forces also have a strong impact on internal policy outcomes within nations. Two sets of external forces appear to have affected health policy in Canada and Australia, at least indirectly. These are the international dissemination of ideas and differences in the degree to which the Australian and Canadian economics have been integrated into the world system.

The Dissemination of Ideas

One of the more interesting aspects of the development of health policy is the speed with which ideas have spread from country to country and the extent to which policy makers have attempted to learn from experience and other jurisdictions. This is true both for ideas about what constitutes 'health' and 'health policy' and for ideas about appropriate policies and programs.

Ideas, some would say ideologies, about health have been influenced by changes in medical science. Until the 1940s, policy discussions contained frequent reference to preventive services. War-induced developments in hospital-based procedures and the control of the most serious infectious diseases by the middle of the century led to a focus on high-technology, curative medical services. As discussed in chapter 5, policy emphasis on the provision of acute-care services came under criticism from a variety of sources in the 1970s. This critique was used in Canada and to a lesser extent in Australia to legitimize reduced government funding, especially for the hospital sector. Although there have been differences in the timing and extent of the responses, health policy in most Western countries has been influenced by these changing ideas. Prevention and primary care came back into the health-policy lexicon in the 1970s.

Policy makers in both federations consistently studied and borrowed ideas from schemes operating in other countries. This practice is common to many governments and groups. In the 1920s and 1930s, for example, requests for copies of the reports of the Australian Royal Commission on National Insurance were received from British Columbia, New Zealand, the New Zealand branch of the BMA, Alberta, South Africa, and the Ontario Medical Association. In the 1940s, requests for information about Australian health-policy proposals came from as far afield as Argentina, China, Quebec, British Columbia, Czechoslovakia, and the Saskatchewan State Hospital and Medical League.[7]

The Australian governments of the 1940s were strongly influenced by the policies of their counterparts, the Labour governments of Britain and New Zealand. The Canadian government's Interdepartmental Advisory Committee on Health Insurance examined the health systems in operation in thirty-nine countries during the Second World War. Similarly, the Canadian Royal Commission of the early 1960s and the Castonguay Commission undertook extensive international research. The incomplete coverage and administrative expense of voluntary health insurance in

Australia influenced the royal commission in its decision to recommend compulsory insurance for Canada. Later in the decade, the Nimmo Committee included a number of practices borrowed directly from Canada in its proposals for reform of the Australian system. Delegations of officials from New Zealand visited Australia in 1986 and early 1987 in an attempt to learn from the operation of Medicare.

The dissemination of ideas in Europe has followed a similar pattern. A longitudinal study of health policy in five countries found that 'throughout the development of their national health programs, the survey countries sought to learn from the experience of other countries. This interest in a neighbour's solutions was more intense at times when important changes were being considered. For example, in both England and Wales and in France the introduction of compulsory sickness insurance was accompanied by study and controversy about the system in operation in Germany' (Blanpain 1978: 269).

Thus the spread of ideas has been an important force in health policy, and indications suggest that this trend will continue. Financial, ideological, and political constraints and perhaps cultural and language barriers may have so far militated against the adoption of Quebec reforms in other Canadian jurisdictions. However, in 1982 the introduction of community centres providing both health and social services on the Quebec model was under consideration in France (Rodwin 1982: 315).

The Impact of Integration into the World Economy

Differences between countries in the rate of 'expansion of the public economy,' which encompasses, of course, the development of the modern welfare state, have been explained by a variety of factors internal to countries or groups of countries. The most important of these are levels of economic development, the tendencies towards expansion inherent in policies once in operation, demographic factors, differences in politicial structure and party ideology, differences in taxation arrangements giving rise to more or less visible taxes, and difference in the degree of financial centralization (Wilensky 1965; Castles and McKinlay 1979a, 1979b; Cameron 1978). In the last few years, however, analysts have begun to include international economic factors in their explanations of different national outcomes. Some countries are more dependent than others on external markets, foreign capital, and imported goods. Integrated into the international system, such 'open' economy countries are subject to a range of externally generated economic forces over which national governments have limited control (Cameron 1978: 1249–51). Small countries are particularly vulnerable to fluctuations in international markets and, in order to shield citizens from the consequences of economic vulnerability, such as structural change and unemployment, the governments of these countries have expanded the role of the state to provide a framework of protective social infrastructure. According to Cameron (1978: 1260), 'governments in small open economies have tended to provide a variety of income supplements in the form of social security schemes, health insurance, unemployment benefit, job training, employment, subsidies to firms and even investment capital.' Thus countries with small open economies are likely to have well-developed welfare states. Cameron terms this 'international explanation' of the expansion of the public economy.

However, integration into the world economy accompanied by the development of comprehensive welfare and industry policies is not the only response to the problems faced by small nations with relatively weak economies. Other options include the adoption of neo-mercantilist policies and various kinds and levels of protection (Cameron 1978: 1260). Australia, of course, has adopted the latter solution and, traditionally, has maintained a relatively closed economy.

Drawing on the work of writers such as Cameron (1978) and Katzenstein (1985), Castles has recently examined the development of Australian public policy in the light of these ideas. He argues that instead of adopting policies of 'domestic compensation,' as many small European countries with open economies have done, Australia has instead opted for a 'politics of domestic defence,' the aim of which is to insulate the main economic groups from the uncertainties of exposure to international economic forces. The main mechanisms of 'domestic defence' historically have been tariff protection, centralized wage fixing, control of immigration (the white Australia policy), and a residual social policy. A comprehensive welfare state has not been developed in Australia because the main avenue of protection is through the labour market. Social policy is residual because it is intended primarily for those outside the workforce. Castles (1988: 108) explains the difference between European social democracy and the Australian approach, termed 'labourism,' in the following terms: 'social democratic reformism can readily by seen as an attempt to tame capitalism by compensating the poor and the weak for the inevitable dislocation caused by economic competition, whereas labourism stresses the need to defend the working man [sic] by the economistic strategy of protecting or enhancing the size of his pay packet.'

Different responses to economic vulnerability may be one of the reasons for Canada's commitment to national health insurance being much stronger than Australia's. Both countries have relatively small economies, although as Canada is considerably larger than Australia, its is more difficult to classify (Castles 1988: 42–3). However, whereas Canada's is a relatively open economic system, Australia's became the third-most closed economy among OECD countries in the post-war period (Castles 1988: 41–6; Banting 1990: 4–5). Following the arguments of Cameron and Castles, then, the comparative openness of the Canadian economy is one of the factors facilitating the development of social infrastructure, including national health insurance. In contrast, Australia until recently has resisted integration into the world economy. The 'politics of domestic defence' involves social protection through participation in the labour market rather than by means of comprehensive welfare provision.

Other Policy Determinants

A number of other policy influences must be mentioned briefly. At times, individuals such as Ian Mackenzie, former minister in the British Columbia government that attempted to introduce public health insurance in the 1930s and minister at the federal level in the 1940s, have played key roles. In the 1980s the committment of Monique Bégin appears to have been a crucial factor in the passage of the Canada Health Act. Generally, however, individuals have only been able to influence policy outcomes when they enjoyed support both within and without Cabinet. Sir Earle Page, former surgeon and federal minister for Health in Australia in the 1950s, was an influential figure in Health but he acted in accordance with principles and policies traditionally supported by the non-Labor parties and the medical profession.

Developments in medical science and the associated 'ideology of curative medicine' were important forces in both Canada and Australia, as in all Western countries. Recently, the critique of curative medicine has been used by governments to legitimize expenditure restraint. Budgetary considerations have always been important in health policy, but it was not until the 1970s that the reluctance of governments to continue to finance the rapid expansion of high-cost, hospital-based services became a political issue. This change in orientation has long-term implications for the mix of services that will be provided, and for the nature of medical practice (Weller 1980: 406–9; Opit 1983: 238–46).

This account of health-policy development demonstrates that many complex forces have operated together to produce policy outcomes. The arguments of analysts such as Simeon (1976) and Hawker, Smith, and Weller (1979), who contend that policy studies that focus on one or two variables can provide only incomplete explanations, are thus confirmed. Having examined the main determinants of policy, we can now attempt to assess the importance of the institutions of federalism. The evidence suggests that the orthodox literature seriously overstates the extent to which generalizations about the impact of divided power can be made.

The Role of Federal Institutions

Deadlock and Delay

At the most obvious level, few instances of deadlock and delay were generated by intergovernmental disagreement in the long process of health-policy making. It is true that proposals for health insurance were abandoned in Canada when the provinces refused to agree to the continuation of financial centralization after the end of the Second World War. However, there was little support for social-policy reform among members of the federal Cabinet. The minister who had promoted health insurance at the federal level had been removed from his portfolio a year earlier. He was replaced by Brooke Claxton, who, after retiring from politics, was an active supporter of private insurance. The overwhelming impression is that health was included in the federal package offered to the provinces in order to increase its political attractiveness. Although a joint system of health insurance failed to materialize, the provinces retained the power to proceed without federal assistance, and several exercised the option.

The only example of a complete deadlock occurred in Australia when Queensland refused to terminate its free system of hospital care in the early 1950s. However, Commonwealth policy was implemented in all other states, despite initial resistance. The Whitlam government encountered difficulties in the early 1970s when negotiating hospital agreements with the non-Labor states, but Medibank began operation in all jurisdictions within three months of the scheduled commencement date. The opposition of the medical profession and ideological and party political factors were the main obstacles to agreement. State Health ministers had endorsed a very similar set of arrangements for paying doctors for public hospital work in 1971, but, in 1974–5, non-Labor state governments were initially unwilling to confront the profession on behalf of the Commonwealth government. The lure of federal funds soon induced them to do so, however, and the pressure on the Commonwealth was relieved.

The opposition of provincial governments was a constraint on federal decision making when the Canada Health Act was under consideration. However, through the combined actions of both levels of government, the universal aspects of health insurance were preserved and strengthened. Despite the division of power, or perhaps even partly because of it, the policy outcome can be seen as an example of 'strong' government, since it was achieved in the face of intense medical opposition that included a serious doctors' strike in Ontario. This achievement is the more impressive when we consider that, on the basis of experience in ten (mostly unitary) countries, Marmor and Thomas predicted that governments could not win pay disputes with the medical profession.

The excessive legalism that Dicey and others predicted was not a significant constraint on policy making. There have only been two instances of constitutional challenge in Australia. Both were in the 1940s and both concerned the pharmaceutical-benefits scheme. These exercises did not of themselves delay the introduction of policy since the leaders of the BMA staunchly refused to cooperate with the government and the vast majority of the association's members were prepared to abide by the council's advice. In a free society, 'the conscription of labour,' as the issue was portrayed, is unacceptable. Public support for the scheme would have needed to have been very much stronger before the government could have contemplated imposing fines on almost every member of the medical profession. The constitution was a useful avenue through which the BMA could resist government initiatives, but there is nothing to suggest that the policy outcome was thereby changed.

The constitutional challenge to the validity of the Canada Health Act currently being sponsored by the Canadian Medical Association has the potential to alter the federal balance of power in relation to responsibility for health. However, even if the challenge is successful, it will be some time before the implications for the health-care system become apparent.[8] Apart from these relatively infrequent instances, there are few cases of obstruction that can be attributed to the institutions of federalism. In general, whenever governments have been firmly committed to action, their policy objectives were realized, except in circumstances where the cooperation of the medical profession could not be secured.

In fact, the most striking instances of implementation difficulties and failure took place when policy responsibility rested with a single government. The McGowen government of New South Wales was unable to implement its hospital policy between 1910 and 1916. The British Columbia government of the 1930s finally abandoned its proposals for health insurance, two weeks before the scheme was due to begin, because of intense medical and business opposition. The Australian government was unable to implement its medical-service and pharmaceutical-benefits policies in the 1940s because doctors refused to participate, and the Saskatchewan government was forced to compromise with the profession to such an extent that its original policy proposals were abandoned entirely. In contrast, policies that required intergovernmental agreement were successfully implemented in every case, except in Canada in the immediate post-war period. The Australian tuberculosis program and hospital-benefits scheme were brought into operation in the 1940s without controversy or delay. Although there was some federal-provincial conflict, the Canadian national hospital and medical-insurance schemes were successfully implemented. Obstruction was avoided in Canada through processes of negotiation and by political pressure on some provincial governments to provide benefits to citizens.

Cooperation and Conflict

Australian health-policy making demonstrates that, under certain conditions, intergovernmental relations can be amicable and cooperative. The joint policy making of the 1940s was remarkably free of conflict on both questions of federal intervention and on matters of policy. Again in 1983–4, federal–state negotiations proceeded to agreement on the conditions under which Medicare would be introduced with minimal difficulty. The key to these periods of genuine cooperation is party: on both occasions Labor governments held office in most jurisdictions. Similarly, during the termination of Medibank between 1976 and 1981, non-Labor governments predominated. However, even when state governments strongly opposed Commonweatlth policy, as when the hospital cost-sharing agreements were arbitrarily declared invalid, they were nearly powerless in the face of federal financial domination. Nevertheless, despite the many unilateral Commonwealth decisions during this period that profoundly affected state budgets, instances of overt conflict were rare.

Intergovernmental relations in Canada reflect the greater degree of provincial autonomy and the prevalence of the idea that the governments are 'equal in rank with each other' (Tuohy 1989b: 399–402). Competition and conflict between government is at least as important as that between parties. Fox (1982: 320) argues that provincial governments, whatever their 'political stripe,' find it politically advantageous to defend provincial rights against the federal government, especially in areas of taxation, finance, and resources. Thus, the Canadian system is not as conducive to periods of cooperation between governments of the same political persuasion as the Australian system but intense partisan competition plays a less important role. In contrast with Australia, 'dogma is either ignored or soft-pedalled and the provincial governments seek to become all things to all people ... like federal governments, the provincial administrations move according to the inexorable fundamental law of Canadian politics towards the centre of the road or perhaps it would be more precise to say they spread themselves all over the road' (Fox 1982: 320). Degrees of party integration and ideological factors, therefore, have a strong bearing on intergovernmental relations. In Australia but not in Canada, party integration can sometimes override conflict between governments at the two levels of the system and result in high levels of cooperation.

Federalism and Interest Groups

Health policy is a most appropriate area in which to examine the influence of interest groups. However, there is little evidence in Australian and Canadian experience to support the argument that federalism augments the power of groups by multiplying points of access to the processes of policy making. As discussed above, in the two cases where the medical profession was able to completely prevent policies from coming into operation – in British Columbia and in Australia in the post-war period – it negotiated, or, more accurately, refused to negotiate, with a single government. In both cases, the policies being proposed were new, and the profession was supported by the party in opposition. Where governments prevailed despite intense medical opposition, as in Australia in the 1970s and Australia and Canada in the 1980s, policy implementation required action by both levels of government. Indeed a case can be made that suggests that the division of power provided governments with a degree of flexibility that facilitated implementation. The successful operation of programs in some provinces and states increases pressure on the remaining governments to provide the same benefits to citizens and makes it more difficult for the medical profession to argue persuasively that policies to which it is opposed will have detrimental effects. Moreover, federalism allows different governments to employ a variety of methods of gaining the compliance of the profession as was the case at the state level in Australia in 1975. Similarly the government of Canada was able to pass the Canada Health Act, an electorally popular move, but could leave the politically difficult task of implementation to the provinces. As with the introduction of hospital and medical insurance, the provinces were free to decide if and when to respond.

Finally, if federalism divides the power of government, it also divides the power of interest groups. The division of power among the Canadian medical associations reflects the federal division of responsibility for health care. The CMA does not play a major political role: most of the action is taken by provincial associations.[9] To the extent that the provinces are the senior level of government in relation to health, Canada resembles ten unitary systems with ten independent medical associations.

Centralization versus Decentralization

'Orthodox' theories of federalism hold that a high degree of centralization is needed in order to facilitate 'strong' government, a position supported by both major parties in Australia and one that traditionally has been an article of faith within the Labor party. Canadian and early Australian health-policy experience, however, shows that social-democratic programs can be implemented in a highly decentralized system. Moreover, federalism does not prevent radical policies from spreading from jurisdiction to jurisdiction, as Madison thought it would. In Canada's national system of separate provincial schemes, national standards have been established. It is true that there is less policy uniformity when responsibility is decentralized, but it cannot be assumed that policy is less 'developed' as a consequence. The examples of Queensland, Tasmania, Saskatchewan, and Quebec show that regional governments can introduce programs that are more innovative than those under consideration in other jurisdictions. State governments, provincial governments, and both federal governments played important roles in the development of Canadian and Australian health policies. Sometimes these governments acted together, sometimes separately, and at other times in sequence. Whether the sum of this activity resulted in more or less innovation or 'stronger' or 'weaker' government *than would otherwise have been the case* simply cannot be measured.

The centralization of power, as Australian experience clearly shows, can result in outcomes which social democrats appear not to have anticipated. The expanded Commonwealth powers that Labor gained during the 1940s were used by the incoming non-Labor government to institutionalize a system of private insurance and private medical practice antithetical to Labor objectives. When Labor regained office in the 1970s, the federal powers, particularly the federal financial power, facilitated the implementation of Medibank. However, the same powers were used with equal effectiveness by the next government to dismantle public insurance and to reintroduce the voluntary health-insurance system. Thus the evidence from health might support the argument, so strongly promoted by Australian social democrats, that centralization facilitates the implementation of Labor's programs but it does not follow that centralization is an expansionary force in welfare-state development. Both parties are able to impose policies from the centre, but these policies may not survive a change of government. Decentralization might even provide protection for programs in the intensely partisan atmosphere of Australian politics: processes of joint policy development may result in stronger commitment among politicians and bureaucrats at the state level, and efforts to explain and sell policies by state governments may serve to strengthen community support.

To summarize the main findings of this study: political parties, party competition, elections, ideas, ideologies, interest groups, economic factors, and the degree to which public opinion is mobilized – all have been important determinants of Canadian and Australian health policy. Institutions are therefore just one among many factors that may have had a bearing upon policy outcomes. Little concrete evidence has been found to support the theories that suggest that federal institutions give rise to weak, conservative governments hemmed in by legal, constitutional, and political obstacles. Rather, political obstacles have been found to be the overwhelming constraint. Canada has been more successful than Australia in developing and preserving a system of universal health insurance despite the decentralized nature of its federal institutions. Australian experience shows that centralized power can be used to impede as well as promote the development of social policies, depending upon the political persuasion of the party in power. Federalism can give rise to intergovernmental conflict, but at other times there can be high levels of cooperation. Nor need conflict be a restrictive force in terms of innovative policy development: provincial pressure on the Canadian government in the 1950s resulted in an extension of public responsibility for hospital care. The introduction of Medibank in Australia and the elimination of extra-billing in Canada were facilitated by the division of responsibility. A flexible situation was created in which governments were able to use a variety of strategies and were able to manipulate the timing of their responses in the face of intractable medical opposition.

The main difference between recent Australian and Canadian experience appears to be the much higher level of support for social programs such as Medicare in Canada, and, of course, the emergence of, and continued support for, a third political party that promotes welfare-state expansion. The lesson from Canada for Australian social democrats is not that centralization is necessary but rather that the main task at hand is to gain the support of a greater proportion of citizens for a strong welfare sector. Such a change might well be facilitated by decentralization, particularly if efforts were made at the same time to democratize the processes of decision making, which, in most areas of health policy, have been highly secret. The processes through which the AIDS policy and the National Women's Health Policy were formulated in the 1980s may offer appropriate pointers (Gray 1990).

The 'Revisionist' Theory of Federalism

If 'orthodox' theories are an accurate guide to the operation of federal systems, can the 'revisionist' theory be more usefully employed as an explanatory tool? There is much to support Trudeau's thesis in Canadian and early Australian experience. Saskatchewan's pioneering role is a classic example of a radical government that was able to introduce social-democratic policies that then spread to other jurisdictions. The role of Quebec in the elimination of extra-billing is another. Some Australian states introduced health-policy reforms long before such policies were considered at the national level. Government control of hospitals, achieved in Tasmania during the First World War and in Queensland in the interwar period, is still a contested issues between the two major federal parties, but Labor continues to pursue policies based on free public hospitals. Canadian policy development supports Cairn's view that federalism may give rise to the coexistence of a number of activist governments where multiple sets of bureaucratic and political élites compete with one another for power, prestige, and political support. The competitive struggle does seem to have helped create an expansionist dynamic that has led to the growth of government activity in the health sector. The intergovernmental conflict surrounding the passage of the Canada Health Act might be seen as an example of expansionism: the federal government saw an opportunity to enhance its position and support by taking action against unpopular user-charges that were being implemented or tolerated by the provinces. The result is increased government control of the health system.[10]

In a recent study of federalism and Canadian health policy, Tuohy (1989a) finds support for an expansionist dynamic in Canadian federalism. She argues that the changing climate of intergovernmental relations has affected the timing of policy innovations and that the division of responsibility has created opportunities for the introduction of new policies at the provincial level and, at the same time, provided a means for policy diffusion. Her conclusion is that 'it is the accommodation of interests, arising from the interplay of economic and ideological factors, and the logic of the policy challenges which result from this accommodation, which define the range of the possible in Canadian health care policy. The effects of federalism are to allow for a variety of accommodations within this range, and to provide both periodic and on going pressures towards convergence' (1989a: 158).

The 'revisionist' thesis finds partial support in Leman's (1977) comparative study of social-security development in Canada and the United States. Leman found that, whereas a continuous, cumulative pattern of policy evolution is characteristic of Canada, the U.S. pattern is one of 'episodic' development. The fragmentation of power, both at the national level and regionally, is given as the explanation for the 'curious stop and go experience' in the United States. In such a system, pressures for change have to build to crisis proportions before innovation is undertaken. Once enacted, new policies become entrenched because change requires not only that the original obstacles be surmounted all over again but also that the views of the new agency and its clients be considered. Since power is also fragmented in Canada, Leman, of course, finds it puzzling that Canada displays the continuous pattern of development that Heclo's (1974) study of social-policy development in Britain and Sweden found to be characteristic of unitary systems with the capacity for centralized political control and the imposition of policy from above. Two features of Canadian federalism are offered in explanation. First, the system allows third parties to gain a 'parliamentary foothold' and thus a platform for proposals in the regions and, second, divided jurisdiction creates the prospect of deadlock so that policy makers urgently seek compromise in order to avert a crisis that might threaten the stability of the federation. The latter dynamic, according to Leman, operates to prevent radical innovation, and promotes continuous, incremental policy adjustment. Thus, in terms of the 'revisionist' thesis, divided jurisdiction has both contractionary and expansionary effects. The regional foothold available to third parties, however, can be a strongly expansionist force. Leman (1977: 275) attributes the introduction of aged pensions to 'a tiny party, a Prime Minister and an impatient province.' Pressure for benefit increases was strong in the 1940s and was directed towards provincial governments that administered and partly funded the program. Leman (1977: 275) argues that 'the provincial governments thus felt pressure from their clients for higher payments, and they transmitted the pressure to the federal government, more effectively perhaps than if the clients had petitioned the federal government directly.'

Leman's study, then, shows that forces similar to those we have seen in health were important in early social-security development. His findings give weight to Trudeau's ideas and partly support a 'revisionist' interpretation.

Evidence of both 'orthodox' and 'revisionist' ideas is also found in Banting's (1987) study of the development of Canadian income security. 'Divided jurisdiction today,' Banting (1987: 82) contends, 'has both a conservative and an expansionist dynamic.' Like Leman, Banting argues that Canadian federalism militates against comprehensive reform but promotes incremental change. The enormous difficulties of extricating the federal variable from the many factors affecting policy are apparent in Banting's study, where generalizations about the impact of federalism are frequently qualified. For example, having noted 'the complexity of conflicts over pensions among business, labour and various social groups,' Banting argues that the fragmentation of decision-making authority was a central factor in the failure to achieve radical pension reform in the 1980s. However, he concludes that 'political institutions are never the only factor influencing policy outcomes, and in the early 1980's the economic recession proved equally important in tempering the reformist impulses of governments' (1987: 208). It could be argued equally well that economic recession was the most important constraining influence, an argument that would be supported by the rapidity with which intergovernmental differences were overcome when budgetary concerns became paramount in the course of negotiating the change to Established-Programs Financing in the 1970s. The reality is that it is frequently almost impossible to determine the independent impact of different forces in policy-making processes.

Moreover, Banting's analysis illustrates the difficulties of attempting to make generalizations about the overall impact of federalism, which is, after all, no more than a set of channels through which many other forces are moving. After weighing the evidence in relation to to the conservative and expansionist theses, he concludes: 'whether divided jurisdiction is, on balance, a conservative or expansionist force in income security, or whether the two sides are broadly self-cancelling, is more difficult to judge ... perhaps ... the benefit of the doubt should be given to the conservative side. The impact, however, is not overwhelming' (1987: 76).

Overall, Banting does not give the benefit of the doubt to the conservative side, but in the final sections of the work a new idea is introduced, which, with other features of Canadian federal politics, could be used to support a 'revisionist' interpretation. The fragmentation of power, Banting argues, that operates to prevent radical expansion of welfare policies also operates to prevent radical retrenchment in response to neo-conservative ideas and the budgetary pressures. He found that the structure of Canadian federalism and the way in which income security is financed constrained the capacity of the federal government to cut programs in the 1980s. Reduced federal funding negatively affects provincial programs, provincial budgets, and provincial economies. Provincial governments thus respond with hostility and have 'impressive capacities to mobilize wider public opposition' (Banting 1987: 208). Banting found that, in income security, the provinces had not been similarly constrained. However, in health, provincial moves towards privitization were stemmed by demands for federal action and the subsequent passage of the Canada Health Act. Thus, from the various strands of the 'revisionist' thesis, observations from this study, and some of the points raised by Banting and Leman, an argument along the following lines can be cobbled together.

Different regions of a nation are usually at different stages of political, social, and economic development. Federalism allows radical parties to gain a foothold in regions where thinking is conducive to expanded government activity. Innovative programs can thus be introduced more easily than in a unitary system because a national consensus does not need to be fashioned. Regional programs operate as 'pilot projects' and, where successful, demonstrate viability and popularity. Competition between governments for prestige and political support and pressure from citizens for equal benefits promote such expansionism, which increases their power. Citizens at the local level are able to influence regional governments, and national governments need to become involved if their prestige and links with citizens are to be maintained. Regional governments welcome federal financial resources, which they do not have to raise themselves. The strength of opposing groups is undermined because arguments about disastrous consequences are more difficult to establish when a program is operating effectively. Self-interest is readily apparent, and 'other-interest' arguments are more difficult to sustain. Moreover, the strength of regionalism presents a potential threat to the stability of the polity, and interest groups are excluded as governmental and bureaucratic élites seek crisis-averting compromises. New federal and provincial programs that emerge from this process are insulated from retrenchment and termination because cuts by the federal government adversely affect provincial governments while the federal government can increase its prestige and support by opposing the erosion of welfare programs at the regional level. Thus, on balance, federalism operates as an expansionary force in welfare-state development.

There is much in Canadian social-policy development that supports this revisionist scenario. Health-policy experience fits the thesis remarkably well, as do early initiatives in income-security development. Legal aid is another policy area where provincial initiatives, particularly in Saskatchewan and Quebec, were taken up in other jurisdictions and where provincial pressure led, first, to federal funding for criminal legal aid, then to cost-sharing of civil legal aid through the Canadian Assistance Plan (Gray, in press). The problem with the revisionist theory, however, is that it cannot be applied to Australian health or social-policy experience in the post-war period. Constrained by federal occupation of the health-insurance field and by their financial dependence on the Commonwealth, the states, far from experimenting and initiating, struggled to meet an increasing share of escalating hospital costs and to develop services to fill glaring gaps in their health systems. In legal aid, repeated calls from the states and the legal profession throughout the 1960s for federal financial support for embryonic state programs met with a negative response. When the Whitlam government came to power, a national legal-aid program, seemingly the brain-child of a single individual, Attorney General Lionel Murphy, was imposed from the centre with no prior discussion. In the characteristic Australian pattern, this program was wound down and handed back to the states by the next non-Labor government. Nor is there evidence of an expansionist dynamic in Australian federalism in relation to income security, at least since the Commonwealth entered the field in 1908. In aged pensions, for example, three states introduced radically progressive schemes in response to demands that arose during the recession of the 1890s. The Commonwealth was given concurrent power for aged and invalid pensions in the Constitution of 1901 and, in 1908–9, a national, tax-financed, means-tested program was introduced that superseded state schemes. Despite non-Labor proposals to introduce contributory insurance in the 1920s, the 1930s, and the early 1950s, Labor promises of a national scheme in the 1970s and 1980s, and sporadic campaigns for the abolition of the means test, the original scheme has operated virtually unchanged since its inception eight decades ago. The one significant reform, abolition of the means test for people aged seventy and over, introduced by the Whitlam government, was partly abolished by the incoming Fraser government. Perhaps the most characteristic feature of the Australian welfare state in recent decades is its reversibility.

The problems of applying Leman's findings about Canada and the United States to the Australian social-security case would form the basis of an interesting study but cannot be explored here. It is sufficient to note that Australia's income-security experience is entirely different from that of Canada and the United States *and* from that of Britain and Sweden: decades of stagnation have prevailed despite almost totally centralized policy responsibility.

Alan Cairns's work is primarily concerned with an analysis of the dynamics of Canadian federalism. Since intergovernmental competition in Australia, when it emerges, largely takes the form of partisan conflict rather than rivalry for prestige and policy space, it is not surprising that Australian experience provides little support for his ideas. Throughout the 1950s and 1960s levels of intergovernmental conflict in Australia were low. The Commonwealth had achieved an unchallenged position as the senior level of government, and academics paid scant attention to state politics during this period. Indeed, to the extent that the states were discussed at all, they were seen by many as 'little more than administrative agencies of the commonwealth, with little money, little will, and little skill' (Davis 1987: 22). There was therefore little reason to oppose their abolition, a proposal made by some academics and a number of Labor leaders, including Gough Whitlam.

With the election of the Whitlam government in 1972, there was, not surprisingly in view of the prime minister's attitudes to federalism, a sharp increase in intergovernmental conflict. Although frequently couched in the rhetoric of states' rights, much of this conflict was of a party political nature. It cannot be seen as a competition among governments to augment their status and power through the occupation of as many policy fields as possible because non-Labor state governments frequently opposed an expanded role in health- and social-policy areas on grounds of principle. Moreover, successive non-Labor federal governments, as noted above, have resisted an expansion of responsibility in welfare areas. The partisan nature of much of Australian intergovernmental conflict is illustrated by the approach of the former non-Labor premier of Queensland, Sir Joh Bjelke-Petersen, who strongly opposed both Medibank and Medicare, even though a system that was very similar, despite different financing arrangements, had operated in his state since the 1940s.

After the defeat of Labor in 1975, intergovernmental conflict again subsided. The period of Fraser government was one of non-Labor dominance in most jurisdictions, and Labor has held the lion's share of office during the period of the present Hawke regime. Garth Stevenson, in discussion with the author, has suggested that federal arrangements in Australia may represent the worst of all possible federal worlds: the states are strong enough to create political difficulties for the Commonwealth but may be too weak to take initiatives themselves. While this insight highlights the very different dynamics of Australian and Canadian federalism, it should be qualified: health-policy experience shows that the power of the states to frustrate federal initiatives is severely limited by their lack of financial autonomy. With the single exception of Queensland in the 1950s, Commonwealth governments of both political persuasions have consistently achieved their objectives throughout the post-war period. Australian experience therefore suggests that revisionist ideas are more likely to be relevant in federations where regionalism is strong and where regional governments enjoy a high level of financial independence. The 'revisionist' thesis does not apply and therefore lacks universal applicability. Trudeau, Cairns, and Banting are writing not about the dynamics of federalism but rather about the dynamics of Canadian federalism.

Health Policy in International Perspective

From this study, generalizations can be made about the way two federal systems operate and about the implications of greater or lesser degrees of centralization. Strictly speaking, however, generalizations cannot be made about similarities and differences between federal and unitary systems. Although there is little evidence of weak, beleaguered government, Canadian and Australian experience needs to be compared with that of similar unitary systems in order to provide a check on the overall impact of federal arrangements. A review of health-policy development in unitary systems shows a wide variety of experiences that are difficult to compare, but there is no clear evidence that policy was, or is, more advanced. Early Australian developments shared similarities with those of many European countries, and with New Zealand. Since the Second World War, however, the Australian proclivity for oscillation between free and fee-charging hospital systems and between public and private health insurance is without parallel in other countries, whatever the institutional arrangements. In international terms, government intervention in health was late in Canada. However, in the 1980s, the level of government responsibility for the financing and organization of the health system is comparable with that of most unitary countries. Canadians have rejected the privatization policies being pushed in many unitary systems, and all citizens have access to comprehensive care without charge at the point of service.

Government sponsored or subsidized health insurance was introduced first in imperial Germany in 1883, followed by Denmark in 1892, Belgium in 1890, Britain and Switzerland in 1911, France in 1930, the Netherlands in 1941, Italy in 1942, and Sweden in 1955 (Maynard 1975; Fulcher 1974). The main purpose of intervention was to increase access to services by lowering the cost to patients. In most European countries, intervention took the form of subsidization and regulation of private funds or friendly societies, and, initially, only low-income groups were covered. Gradually, benefits and eligibility were extended in order to provide coverage for most of the population, a process that took many decades. At the same time, government provision or subsidization of hospital and other health services grew steadily.

Australian experience follows that of several unitary countries such as Britain, New Zealand, Sweden, and Denmark in the development of a strong public hospital system in the nineteenth and twentieth centuries. Compared with many European countries, Australia was late in developing health insurance, but, like Sweden, which was also very late, the public provision of services was extensive (Blanpain 1978: 169–206). Similarly, in New Zealand, where public health insurance has never been introduced, there has been heavy reliance on the direct provision of services. Both Australia and New Zealand, following British ideas, attempted to establish national health services in the 1940s. Hospital care was made universally available and free in both countries but, whereas Australia failed to introduce a national medical service because the medical profession was strongly united and refused to cooperate, New Zealand partly succeeded (Condliffe 1959: 304–15). As discussed in chapter 3, however, the relative success of the British and New Zealand governments in the 1940s compared with that of Australia was a result of deep divisions within the respective medical professions. These divisions notwithstanding, both the British and New Zealand governments were forced to make substantial concessions in response to medical demands concerning methods of remuneration. It should be remembered, too, that while Britain was well ahead of Australia in introducing public subsidies for health insurance, the coverage of the 1911 scheme, which operated until 1948, was very limited. Only low-income workers were covered, and benefits did not extend to dependents. In contrast, Australian friendly-society schemes covered all family members. Prior to the Second World War, Australian and British Columbian experience in relation to health insurance is similar to that of the Netherlands, where several policy proposals were defeated by the medical professions. Insurance was finally imposed in the Netherlands in 1941 by the German occupation forces (Blanpain 1978: 129–33).

Compared with Europe, Australia, and New Zealand, governments in North America were slow to intervene in the health sector, in relation to both health insurance and direct service provision. By the Second World War, most Western countries had provided at least low-income citizens with access to a reasonably comprehensive range of services. Thus, it would seem that, in relation to health, Canada is a welfare-state 'laggard.' However, Banting (1987: 31–6) disagrees with this view. He argues that, 'in terms of the socio-economic preconditions of welfare development, Canada's progress was typical or even a little "early."'

Although Banting's argument is persuasive, it cannot explain why government intervention in Canada took place much later than in Australia and New Zealand, where industrial development also lagged behind that of Europe. An additional explanatory factor is needed, and it appears to be that different ideas were dominant in Canada. Australia and New Zealand followed British trends in the development of extensive public sectors in the health area whereas Canada did not. The idea that services, particularly hospital services, should be free for all citizens was a forceful one in Australia and New Zealand, perhaps supporting the Hartz thesis that the origins of political culture do have long-term importance. However, the fact that government intervention was late in Canada, even by non-European standards, does not establish federalism as the cause. Australia developed along European lines, despite its federal constitution. The suggestion here is that the main reason for non-intervention in Canada was the very different set of attitudes towards the provision of health care, which, as discussed in chapter 3, Burdett discovered in North America in the 1890s.

Canadian governments may have been late entrants into the health-policy field, but in terms of achieving the original objective of intervention – that of removing the financial barriers that prevent people from receiving care – they have been very successful in recent decades. The long process through which other countries, both unitary and federal, gradually extended access to a more comprehensive range of services and to greater numbers of citizens was cut short. Among OECD nations in the 1980s, Britain is the other country that provides universal access to hospital and medical services without charge. User-charges, even modest ones, have been shown to restrict service use, especially for the old and the poor. In some countries, such as France, patient co-payments for hospital and medical care are substantial. User charges were introduced or increased in Belgium and Germany in the 1980s, and privatization is on the agenda in Britain, where the private sector of medical practice is expanding in response to new government subsidies (OECD 1985: 63–7; *Independent* 27 January 1989). In New Zealand, hospital services are still free, but much of the social protection provided by the general medical benefit has been lost over the years, as governments have allowed inflation to erode its value. In 1986, benefits covered only 20 to 30 per cent of medical fees, and further privatization is on the political agenda.[11]

In summary, although certain broad patterns can be discerned, health policy in OECD countries evolved in a variety of ways over a very long period of time (doctors' fees, for example, were first regulated in Denmark in 1619). There are important differences between unitary nations, between federations, and between federal and unitary countries. But Canadian and Australian services compare favourably with those of most unitary countries and, where government intervention was late, as in Canada, it is not clear that federalism was the reason. In the 1980s, the trend in many unitary countries and in the United States is towards privatization in the health sector. Paradoxically, perhaps, Canada and Australia are currently moving against the international tide.

Theories of Federalism?

The findings of this study strongly suggest that attempts to develop a general theory of the impact of federalism on the scope of government activity are likely to be frustrated by insurmountable problems. The institutions of federalism operate in very different social, political, economic, and cultural settings. Canada and Australia share a great many common features, yet the institutions and politics of the two systems are markedly different. The problems of developing a theory of the operation of two like systems are multiplied and magnified if unlike systems such as those of India and Malaysia are included. Moreover, arrangements within single federations change both over time and in response to the many fluctuating forces within political systems. Clearly, any theory of Australian or Canadian federalism developed early in the life of either system would need now to be substantially revised to accommodate significant changes in the balance of power.

These problems are addressed in a recent work on the federal principle that is subtitled *A Journey through Time in Quest of a Meaning*. Federalism is a concept that has 'lived a long life,' Davis (1978: ix) notes, but it is one that is beginning 'to show distinct marks of wear and tear.' The problems of studying federalism, he argues, are apparent in the development of many different approaches to the subject and in repeated efforts to clarify the meaning of the term.

Although more is known about the subject than ever before, Davis argues, theories of federalism have become 'less satisfying' and 'less reputable.' He lists more than half a page of adjectives, ranging from 'peripheralized' to 'unitary' and from 'competitive' to 'feudal-functional,' that have been coined to try to add precision to the meaning of the concept. He suggests that the confusion arises because the study of federalism involves the study of things that 'are only partly the same.' If there is a 'logic' that is common to all federations, 'it lacks the force to transcend their different political cultures and impose a common political direction' (1978: 204–12).

Davis's contentions are borne out by this comparison of the operation of the Australian and Canadian federations. Differences in the division of constitutional and financial power, in the degree of party integration, in the levels of cultural homogeneity, and in ideas and ideologies have resulted in contrasting policy processes and considerable variation in policy outcomes. The fact that there are many similarities between the two systems of health care in the mid-1980s cannot be attributed to the impact of institutions in which there is so much variation, but is rather the result of forces common to the two countries. These include the international dissemination of ideas, the influence of Canadian experience on some Australian policy makers, similar medical technologies, the success of the medical profession in ensuring the preservation of a large private sector of medical practice in both countries, and some convergence in ideas about what constitutes appropriate access to health care.

However, the similarities between the two systems of insurance may not persist. A change of government at the Commonwealth level in Australia will almost certainly result in extensive privatization in health and other social-policy areas. This change is all the more likely because some leaders of the Right faction in the present Labor government have consistently promoted privatization, without notable success as yet, except in tertiary education. Reprivatization would emerge from the interplay of an array of political forces that would be channelled through existing institutions. On the basis of past experience, it is possible to try to predict the kinds of policies that political parties and the medical profession might promote. It is also possible to try to predict the responses of other groups, and of health consumers in general. But it is almost impossible to predict the independent effect of federal institutions. In the first place, as Simeon (1976: 575) and others have observed, institutions have no policy content of their own: their importance lies 'in the way in which they interact with other social forces.' Second, institutions are only one of the many variables that give rise to distinctive policy processes and policy outcomes. Which variables or set of variables will be the more important in particular cases cannot be foretold. In Australia in the 1940s, for example, the federal division of power was not an important constraint on policy making. The main reason that government objectives were not achieved was the medical profession's refusal to cooperate. However, the division of responsibility in Canada in the 1980s gave rise to intense intergovernmental conflict. As well, although the policy choices open to both levels of government were thereby limited, the medical profession was unable to exert enough influence to achieve its aims. Finally, and importantly, it might be possible to speculate about some of the implications of Australian federalism or Canadian federalism for future policy. It seems plausible to argue, for example, that, in the short term at least, the Commonwealth will continue to dominate Australian health policy, whereas in Canada the provinces will continue to play the more powerful role. But a quite different 'theory' would be needed for each federation. Moreover, in order to attempt to predict the policy outcomes, one would need information about other forces and influences, such as the political persuasion of the parties in power and the level of public support for the position taken by the medical profession. Clearly, such speculation cannot constitute a theory of federalism, or even two theories of federalism – one for Canada and another for Australia.

There appear to be three main reasons that theories of federalism have failed to provide an adequate account of the operation of the Canadian and Australian systems of government, at least in relation to health-policy development. The first is the influence of U.S. experience. By almost any criteria, the United States is a welfare-state 'laggard.' In health policy in particular, it is the only OECD country in which millions of low-income earners still have no coverage against the cost of basic hospital and medical services. Since the universe of comparable federations is so small, consisting of only five nations, the U.S. experience can distort cross-national comparisons. The second reason is that too much weight has been attributed to the influence of just one of the many complex forces that operate in the processes of formulating and implementing public policy. The third is that the distinction between federal and unitary systems has been exaggerated. As several writers have observed, 'federalness' is a matter of degree. The division of responsibility for Canadian health policy is similar in many ways to that of Sweden, where local government has a high level of financial independence and extensive scope for independent decision making within the parameters set by the national government. In contrast, Australian policy, like that of Britain and New Zealand, has been primarily determined by the central government since the Second World War. Thus, institutionally, health-policy-making processes in Canada and Australia may have less in common with each other than they have with some unitary systems of government.

Notes

CHAPTER 1: Federalism and the Study of Public Policy

1 For a discussion of the empirical evidence on this issue see Neumann (1957: 216–29). His conclusion is that federalism, as such, has no inherent features that automatically guarantee the preservation of political freedom.

2 Cameron's findings from his study of eighteen OECD countries do not support an institutional explanation of the expansion of the public economy. Rather, expansion was most closely associated with small national economic size and high levels of dependence on international trade.

3 The literature of public-policy analysis is reviewed by Helco (1972, 1974: 6–9); Simeon (1976); Hawker, Smith, and Weller (1979: 6–26); and Davis, Wanna, Warhurst, and Weller (1988). Castles and McKinlay (1979) provide an overview of the literature that posits environmental explanations of policy outcomes. Theories and models of policy making are discussed by Leach and Stewart (1982), Doern and Phidd (1983), Hill and Bramley (1986), and Davis, Wanna, Warhurst, and Weller (1988).

4 For an extended methodological criticism of comparative studies of Canada and Australia, see Kellow (1988: 59–72).

5 A study of federal and unitary systems designed according to the 'most similar systems' approach could not show with certainty that the federal variable accounted for discovered differences unless the countries being examined were alike in every other way. In practice, sets of such countries are very hard to find. A comparative study of Britain and Australia or Britain and Canada, for example, would fit the 'most similar systems' design very well, but the federal/unitary distinction is by far from the only important difference. A comparative study of the development of public health insurance in Britain and Australia might conclude that federalism is the

reason that Australian developments were many decades behind those in Britain. But many other explanations are possible, such as the Australian Labor party's rejection of contributory insurance or Britain's much earlier industrialization. To complicate the matter further, if New Zealand, another similar system, were included in such a study, a non-institutional reason would have to be found to explain why that country has not so far introduced public health insurance.

CHAPTER 2: The Development of National Health Insurance in Canada, 1900–70

1 For a detailed study of political, economic, and social developments on the prairies, see Lipset (1950).
2 Interview, Mr Chestly Adams, Prince Albert, 22 November 1985
3 Proceedings, Federal-Provincial Conference, 1950
4 Proceedings, Dominion-Provincial Conference, 1957, p. 66
5 Interview, Dr Orville Hjertaas, 22 November 1985. The largest of these clinics or community health centres, which employs about eighteen doctors, also provides a wide range of non-medical health services. It is equipped to perform minor surgery and is located in Prince Albert, where the State Hospital and Medical League was formed in the 1930s. It was in this city that Prime Minister Mackenzie King lost his seat in the 1945 election.
6 A detailed account of the mediation process is given by Lord Taylor in a four-part series published by the CMA Journal in 1974 (110 [23 March 1974, 6 April 1974, 20 April 1974, 4 May 1974]).
7 The Medical Care Act (1967) stipulated that charges to patients at the point of service should not be large enough to deter the use of services (Brown 1984: 19). Thus, there are usually said to be five principles of Medicare or 'national standards': comprehensiveness, universality, portability, public administration, and accessibility (National Council of Welfare 1982: 14–15).
8 The changes that took place in Quebec, often referred to as the Quiet Revolution, will be discussed more fully in chapter 7.
9 This conflict, which led to the passage of the Canada Health Act, 1984, is examined in chapter 5.

CHAPTER 3: Health Services in Australia: White Settlement to 1950

1 The government of Quebec is an exception. Quebec innovations are discussed in chapter 7.
2 The importance of contract practice is discussed in chapter 4.

3 The association was known by this name until 1962 when it became the Australian Medical Association. A federal committee was formed in 1912 and a federal council in 1933.

4 *MJA* 5 September 1914: 235; 29 May 1915: 510–11; 9 December 1916: 508–9; 9 June 1917: 488–9; 20 October 1917: 335–6; 9 November 1918: 394

5 For an account of hospital construction and improvement and the expansion of public health services in the mid-1930s, see Ogilvie (1938: 57–64).

6 Leggett provides a detailed account of Queensland health politics in the first half of the century. For a history of the BMA in Queensland, see Robin (1966).

7 Report of the Social Security Medical Survey Committee 1 (1943): 118, 127

8 Policy making during this period has been discussed in some detail by Hunter (1963, 1966, and 1968), by McGrath (1975), and, less extensively, by Thame (1974). These authors have concentrated on the politics of medical opposition, but the federal–state aspects of policy making, which will be the focus of the remainder of this chapter, are discussed only briefly.

9 For a more detailed account of these developments, see Hunter (1968: 136–59).

10 Report of the NHMRC, 11th Session, July 1941: 2; 12th Session, November 1941: 13–43

11 Quoted in Report of the NHMRC, 12th Session, November 1941: 18–19

12 As late as the early 1950s, the states had money set aside for capital expenditure that they were unable to use. In 1947, many tuberculosis beds remained unoccupied because of a shortage of nurses.

13 The tuberculosis scheme is omitted from this list but will be included in discussion below because it was a joint federal–state program.

14 The meaning is 'one-doctor towns.'

15 A successful prototype was in operation in Yallourn, Victoria, and was initiated by the State Electricity Authority for its workers. Non-employees were eligible for membership, and most townspeople had chosen to join. A committee of the JCSS had found that industrial areas were undersupplied with doctors.

16 Cabinet Submission, 16 November 1954, Australian Archives (AA) ACT CRS A1928, Item 100/1, Section 3

17 AA ACT CRS A1658, Item 812/5/2, Section 1

18 AA ACT CRS A1658, Item 813/1/1, Section 1

19 AA ACT CRS A1658, Item 812/5/2, Section 1

20 AA ACT CRS A1658, Item 813/1/1, Section 1

21 AA ACT CRS A1658, Item 813/5/2, Section 1

22 It is at least as likely that few people understood the issues involved. In the 1970s, during a period of frequent health policy changes, up to 40 per cent

of people did not know whether they supported new arrangements or not (Gray 1982: 52).

23 AA ACT CRS A1928, Item 195/239

24 *Minutes of Proceedings of Conference of Ministries for Health of the Commonwealth and States of Australia*, 6 July 1944

25 Victoria, in contrast, stood to gain more than any other state. All states would be relieved of the administrative costs of collecting fees.

26 AA ACT CRS A1658, Item 688/1/1, Section 1

27 Ibid.

28 Tasmania opposed the public subsidization of private patients.

29 *Minutes of Proceedings of Conference of Ministers for Health of the Commonwealth and States of Australia*, 6 May 1946

30 *Conference of Ministers for Health of the Commonwealth and States*, June 1943, July 1944; AA ACT CRS A1658, Item 688/1/1, Section 1

31 Indeed, Tasmanian experience, like that of Saskatchewan, demonstrates that large, wealthy states and provinces are not necessarily policy leaders. Tasmania is the smallest, poorest Australian state, but the level of social-welfare expenditure in the 1940s was 'very much higher than that in any other state' (*Minutes of the Conference of Ministers for Health of the Commonwealth and States of Australia* 1948: 13–14).

32 In another case of the 'demonstration effect,' this was partly based on existing New Zealand legislation.

33 The negotiations between the Commonwealth and the medical profession in the 1940s have been documented in detail by McGrath (1975: 423–539) and by Hunter (1968). McGrath takes a generous view of the degree to which the BMA was prepared to cooperate with the government.

34 At this time, the idea of a national health system based on fee-for-service was new in Australia. Chief promoter of the idea, Dr Charles Byrne of Victoria, who published a book outlining a national system based on this method of remuneration in 1943, was present at the meeting.

35 AA ACT CRS A1928, Item 690/39, Section 6

36 Ibid.

37 *Minutes of the Conference of Ministers for Health of the Commonwealth and States of Australia*, May 1947: 5–33

38 For the BMA's objections and a résumé of the parliamentary debates on the act, see *MJA* 5 February 1949: 159–83. This issue also contains copies of correspondence between the minister and Federal Council.

39 Prime Minister Chifley's letter, informing the BMA that the introduction of the scheme could not be delayed by 'interminable discussion,' is reprinted in *MJA* 16 April 1949: 523–4.

CHAPTER 4: Voluntary Health Insurance in Australia, 1950–72

1 For a history of friendly societies in Australia, see Green and Cromwell (1984). This work documents the long struggle between the societies and the medical profession, known as the 'battle of the lodges.' Sir Earle Page, former surgeon, who became Minister for Health in 1949, had been involved in a 'withdrawal of services' from a Grafton society prior to his entry into parliament. See also Pensabene (1980).

2 Whereas in Australia the medical profession appears to have been united, British specialists had refused to support general practitioners in their campaign to break the power of friendly societies. Many general practitioners thus welcomed national insurance (at the right price) because the government and not the societies determined conditions of service. Specialists also supported the system because it was thought that it would institutionalize general practice and reduce the competition between general practitioners and specialists for hospital appointments. A detailed account of the divisions within the British profession and the influence of these divisions on the type of health system that emerged is given in Honigsbaum (1979).

3 Most of these recommendations were implemented over time, although in a 'haphazard and inconsistent fashion' (Sax 1984: 38).

4 The implementation of these proposals would have given Queensland a health system very similar to the British National Health Service of 1948.

5 AA ACT CRS A1928, Item 625/A/8

6 *Report of the Social Security Medical Survey Committee* (1 [June 1943])

7 Private hospitals contained 26 per cent of total bed capacity in 1941–2. The Medical Survey Committee was unable to establish the number of non-public beds in public hospitals but found that these were 'a small proportion' of the total. In 1952, 80 per cent of hospital patients were public patients in New South Wales so that it can be estimated that roughly 60 per cent of hospital patients were charged no medical fees.

8 The policy, BMA president Sir Victor Hurley argued, was 'submitted as a national necessity and was entirely free from political implications' (BMA 1949: 6).

9 *Official Report of the Fifth Commonwealth Conference of the Australian Labor Party* 1912: 22

10 *Report on Health and Pensions Insurance* (1937: 29)

11 For a detailed account of the formulation and abandonment of the highly controversial National Health and Pensions Insurance Bill of 1938, see Watts (1983: 94–219).

12 Earle Page Papers, National Library of Australia, MS 1633/1346

13 Cabinet Submission, No 16A, 25 January 1950; AA ACT CRS A 1658, Item 669/1/1, Section 1

14 Cabinet Submission, No 16C, 17 April 1950; Earle Page Papers, National Library of Australia, MS 1633/2153

15 AA ACT CRS A1658, Item 669/1/16

16 AA ACT CRS A1658, Item 666/3/4, Section 1

17 In 1962, it was erroneously stated in an article in the MJA that lodge agreements were cancelled in 1949, after which doctors charged a fee for service (MJA 18 August 1962: 23). Many writers, for example Deeble (1970: 49) and Sax (1984: 60), have accepted this error.

18 AA ACT CRS A1658, Item 669/1/1, Section 1

19 Earle Page Papers, National Library of Australia, MS 1633/2153; AA ACT CRS A1658, Item 669/1/1, Section 1

20 *Minutes of the Conference of Commonwealth and State Ministers for Health*, 15 August 1950: 1–32

21 None of the participants said what kind of compulsory system they had in mind but presumably the British system based on contract practice was intended.

22 *Minutes of the Conference of Commonwealth and State Ministers for Health*, 16 January 1951: 1–28

23 AA ACT CRS A1658, Item 200/3/7, Section 1; A1658, Item 668/14/1, Section 1; A1658, Item 668/14/4, Section 1; A1658, Item 668/14/5; A1658, Item 668/14/7, Section 1; A1658, Item 668/28/1; A1658, Item 668/28/2; A1658, Item 668/28/6

24 AA ACT CRS A1658, Item 668/14/5; A1658, Item 668/14/7, Section 1; A1658, Item 668/28/2

25 AA ACT CRS A1658, Item 668/14/5

26 AA ACT CRS A1658, Item 668/14/5; A1658, Item 668/14/7, Section 1

27 This was not the case, however, in one-doctor towns or in rural and industrial urban areas, which were undersupplied with services, particularly specialist services. Nor was it the case for patients referred to specialists or for pensioners who were eligible only for specialist services provided in the outpatients departments of public hospitals.

28 While there were no rules about minimum benefits levels, there was a rule that the benefit could not exceed 90 per cent of the doctor's fee. This rule was intended to protect doctors against 'frivolous demands by patients' (Sax 1984: 65).

29 The British Medical Association in Australia became independent in 1962 and was known thereafter as the Australian Medical Association (AMA).

30 *Report of the Commonwealth Committee of Inquiry into Health Insurance* (1969)

31 It was later argued by a leading journalist that the major funds had become 'self-perpetuating bureaucracies,' free from government control, with close links with hospital boards and the AMA. The federal government merely provided money to keep the system afloat. See Kewley (1973: 507–8).

32 In 1973–4, a study found that failure to pay health bills was the commonest cause of imprisonment for debt in South Australia (Scotton 1989: 130).

CHAPTER 5: Canadian Health Policy under National Health Insurance, 1970–86

1 *Task Force Reports on the Costs of Health Services* (1969)

2 Although medical insurance had not been introduced in all provinces at this time, about half of the population had some level of private insurance coverage (Hall Report 1964: 727) so that the 'insurance effect' operated prior to the introduction of Medicare.

3 These proposals, which are similar to those put forward in Australia in the 1940s, developed later in Canada. The explanation appears to be the earlier development of the public provision of services in Australia compared with the focus upon the insurance principle in Canada. Australian policy was also influenced by ideas in Britain, where the development of health centres had been discussed since the 1920s.

4 For an excellent discussion of the ethical problems raised by modern medicine, particularly in the face of limited government funding, see the *CMA Journal* 132 (15 February 1984): 446–9.

5 At this time, groups began to emerge in the United States, and to a lesser extent in Canada, that demanded a radical new approach to health policy (Weller 1980: 326–39).

6 The degree of polarization in the British Columbia political system is greater than in the rest of Canada, and in this respect appears to resemble the Australian situation.

7 There were considerable variations between the provinces in the types of policies undertaken and also some variation in the degree to which the provinces succeeded in controlling costs. For example, British Columbia tried to reduce the number of doctors in the province by restricting the issue of billing numbers, while Ontario and Quebec were the most successful in reducing the supply of acute care beds. See Barer and Evans (1984).

8 The provisions of this act also apply to the federal government's share of payments for post-secondary education.

9 This is the reason that some of the provinces wanted the federal-government contribution in the form of tax points rather than cash. A tax point is equal to one percentage point of personal income taxation or corporate taxation

and may be adjusted to achieve equalization objectives. When a transfer of tax points takes place, the federal government agrees to reduce its taxation yield by a given number of points. This 'tax room' is then used by a province to raise its own revenue.

10 Negotiations in relation to financial arrangements for social policies do not necessarily coincide with the five-year revision of financial arrangements, but in this case they did.

11 The provinces had, however, put together what was presented to the federal government as a 'consensus' position (Brown 1984: 29).

12 This strategy has been far more successful than attempts to close 'unnecessary' hospitals, which, even where successful, entailed high political costs. For an account of Ontario's cost-containment policies in the 1970s and early 1980s, see Vayda and Deber (1985).

13 *Parliamentary Task Force on Federal Provincial Fiscal Arrangements* (Breau Report) (1981: 100)

14 The term 'extra-billing' was usually used when physicians stayed within the medical plan, i.e., sent their bills to the plan but charged the patient an additional fee. The term 'opting-out' was used when physicians billed the patient directly at, or above, the schedule fee. Thus 'opted-out' doctors may have engaged in extra-billing but did not necessarily do so. A few doctors, for reasons of principle, had never 'opted in,' but charged no more than the schedule fee. In Quebec, as we saw in chapter 2, the patients of an 'opted-out' doctor could not claim reimbursement from the insurance plan, with the result that few doctors chose this path. In most other provinces, direct-billed patients were reimbursed by the plan at the rate of 90 per cent of the schedule fee. The terms 'balance-billing' and 'double-billing' were also used to denote the practice of billing both the plan and the patient.

15 In fact, because of equalization arrangements, cost-sharing had never worked this way, but apparently this was not widely understood by politicians (Brown 1984: 52–3).

16 The Liberal party was not in power in any province between 1978 and 1985. The Parti Québécois governed in Quebec, and Social Credit was in office in British Columbia. The NDP was defeated in 1982 by the Conservative party in Saskatchewan. The Conservative party was in power in all other provinces.

17 Interview, Mr Alex Conolly, 10 October 1985

18 Interview, Mme Bégin, 23 October 1985

19 Interviews: Mr Guy Bujolt, 11 October 1985; Mrs Sheena Lee, 17 October 1985; Mrs Margaret Mitchell, 9 October 1985

20 The alternative view, put forward in the Breau Report the following year,

was that the federal contribution comprised both tax points and the cash grant. It was argued that the provinces had financed virtually all the 'real' expansion of services from federal funds, leaving provincial funds free for use elsewhere. The arguments are complex, involving the question of the actual value of transferred tax points in a time of economic recession. All that can be said with certainty is that, after EPF, the rate of growth of federal funding was faster than that which the provinces found necessary (or chose) to spend from their own sources.

21 Interview, Mr Don McNaught, 17 October 1985
22 Interviews: Mme Bégin, 23 October 1985; Mr Guy Bujolt, 11 October 1985
23 Interview, Mme Bégin, 23 October 1985
24 Interview, Mme Bégin, 23 October 1985. Antagonisms between the provinces and the medical profession over fees and funding levels meant that there was no possibility of a coalition of opposition against the federal government.
25 Opposition to extra-billing and user-charges increased after the federal government took action. In May 1984, 83 per cent of Canadians opposed extra-billing, with only 13 per cent in favour; 68 per cent were opposed to user-charges, with 24 per cent in favour.
26 Interview, Mme Bégin, 23 October 1985
27 Part of the explanation for this change may be that as oil prices fell, many people who had come with the boom left the province. The period of high wages and incomes had passed.
28 Interview, Mr Tim Lynch, 1 November 1985
29 Interview, The Hon. Steven Paproski, Member for Edmonton North, 21 August 1986
30 In July 1986, extra-billing in New Brunswick amounted to an estimated 0.1 per cent of the health budget (*Globe and Mail* 12 July 1986: A3). The government and the profession reached an agreement to eliminate the practice in 1987.
31 Interview, Mr Don MacNaught, 17 October 1985

CHAPTER 6: Compulsory Health Insurance in Australia, 1972–86

1 The policy relating to reform and expansion of health services, which became the responsibility of a separate commission, is discussed in the next chapter.
2 Dental treatment was to be made more freely available to schoolchildren through the expansion of publicly provided services rather than by subsidizing the cost of private services. New Zealand provided a model.

3 Pensioner Medical Service

4 Most of the information for the following sections on the politics of the Whitlam period was obtained from the office files of the then minister for Social Security, The Hon. W.G. Hayden. Quoted with permission

5 Interview, Dr J. S. Deeble, 23 October 1986

6 *The Australian Health Insurance Program* (November 1973: 13–19) (The White Paper)

7 Interview, Dr J. S. Deeble, 23 October 1986

8 Of the estimated gains to the states arising from the new arrangements, the Queensland share was $66 million in a total of $183 million.

9 Mr Hayden became treasurer in the middle of the year but retained responsibility for finalizing the hospital negotiations.

10 Interview , Dr S. Sax, 21 October 1986

11 Health minister Alan Scanlan had supported fee-for-service in line with AMA policy (Sax 1984: 118).

12 Interview, Dr S. Sax, 21 October 1986

13 For more detailed accounts of the termination process, see Sax (1984: 127–83) and Gray (1984).

14 Non-Labor in opposition had been able to prevent Labor from introducing a levy of 1.25 per cent by voting against the necessary legislation in the Senate.

15 Interview, The Hon. Michael MacKellar, MP, 15 June 1982

16 About 5 per cent of Australian doctors are members of this society, which supports universal health insurance and reform of the health-care delivery system.

17 Mr Hayden (currently the Governor General of Australia) was leader of the opposition between 1977 and 1983.

18 Interview, Dr J. S. Deeble, 23 October 1986

CHAPTER 7: Health Services in Canada and Australia, 1970–86

1 In the federal–Quebec bargaining process, Quebec was not able to achieve all of its demands. Ottawa retained control over many aspects of income security, but it was agreed that social policies were to be a provincial responsibility (Coleman 1984: 136–8).

2 *Report of the Commission of Enquiry on Health and Social Welfare*, Vols 1–7 plus appendices

3 In the late 1970s, the payment of cash benefits was transferred to the Department of Manpower and Income Security. The Ministry of Social Affairs was

renamed the Ministry of Health and Social Services in 1984, but its responsibilities were not changed.

4 Interview, Mr Pierre Roberge, 22 October 1985

5 Interview, Dr Jacques Brunet, 21 and 22 October 1985

6 Interview, Dr Gaetan Garon, 22 October 1985

7 Interview, Dr Jacques Brunet, 21 October 1985

8 Interviews: Mrs Sandra Golding, 25 October 1985; Mr Pierre Roberge, 22 October 1985

9 Information about CLSC Metro was gained during two visits to the centre, from interviews with Mrs Sandra Golding, coordinator of the Youth and Women's Clinic, and from the Centre's 1983–4 Annual Report. At 1986 Australian prices, it would cost in the vicinity of $18 million per annum to maintain 950 people in nursing homes.

10 Dr Pineault recognizes that it is perhaps unrealistic to expect that an even faster rate of change might have been achieved during the period of reform (Interview, 25 October 1985).

11 Interview, Dr Jean Denis Dubois, 21 October 1985

12 For a survey of inequalities in health status in Britain, see Townsend and Davidson (1982).

13 Interview, Dr S. Sax, 21 October 1986

14 Ibid.

15 Ibid.

16 Minister for Community Services, News Release, 4 December 1986; Gray (1990)

17 The Department of Community Services and the Department of Health were amalgamated to form a super-ministry, the Department of Community Services and Health, in 1987. The implications of this change need further study, but policy continuity appears to have been maintained.

18 Better Health Commission, *Interim Report* (February 1986: 3)

19 Better Health Commission, *Looking Forward to Better Health* (Vols 1–3, 1986)

CHAPTER 8: Federalism and the Determinants of Health Policy

1 Interview, Mme Bégin, 23 October 1985

2 For a discussion of this literature, see Mayer (1956).

3 Hartz's thesis is that, in the process of founding new societies, single ideologies were detached from their European contexts and implemented in new nations. Whereas, 'there is a process of contagion at work in Europe ... in which ideologies give birth to one another over time,' the fragment is iso-

lated from 'challenges past and future.' The detached ideology is therefore able to flower and unfold, free from competing perspectives (Hartz 1964: 6). The particular ideology cast off depends upon the timing of the settlers' departures from Europe. Thus feudalism was transferred to Latin America and French Canada, Lockean liberalism to British North America, and nineteenth-century British radicalism to Australia. Although the fragment ideology dominates in its new setting, the unfolding process 'works itself out differently in the different fragments.' For example, while English Canada is essentially liberal, it is 'etched with a Tory streak coming out of the American Revolution' (Hartz 1964: 34). English Canada is thus in a sense a fragment thrown off from the United States. The Hartz and Hartz-Horowitz theses have been criticized on many grounds. Preece (1980), for example, questions Horowitz's interpretation of Lockean liberalism, Forbes (1987) finds that developments within French Canada do not fit well with its characterization as a feudal fragment and questions whether Canadian socialism, as represented by the CCF-NDP, is based on 'corporate-organic-collectivist' ideas, as Horowitz claims, or whether it is rather a liberal welfare-state ideology. In Australia, McCarty (1973) and Bolton (1973) both find Hartz's theory of the development of the fragment ideology wanting in that it does not allow for the interaction of environmental influences. Hirst (1984), in contrast, finds support for the Hartz thesis in the Australian eagerness to adopt and adapt British working-class institutions such as mechanics' institutes, friendly societies, and the Labor party in the nineteenth century. Despite their many criticisms and modifications, most of these writers do not dispute that there are important insights in the Hartzian approach and that Horowitz's adaptation draws attention to crucial distinctions between Canadian and US conservatism.

4 Interview, Donald Smiley, 5 November 1985

5 Hartz variously refers to the Australian fragment as 'radical,' 'collectivist,' and 'proletarian' (1964: 4, 7, 16, 43, 51). Hirst (1984: 103–4) argues that the Australian ethos of mutual self-improvement and economic independence is not collectivist but nor is it 'unalloyed individualism.' Similarly, Forbes (1987) has contested Horowitz's categorization of Canadian socialism as 'collectivist.' What can be said, however, is that the left in both Canada and Australia support the use of the power of the democratic state to pursue redistributive policies.

6 After a period in 1987 and 1988, when Medicare appeared to be gaining in support among doctors and the public alike (Gray 1990), opposition began to mount again. The AMA produced a so-called Green Paper, proposing the complete withdrawal of government from health-insurance funding and the

introduction of a system of compulsory private insurance (AMA 1989). The Liberal party has not released a new health-policy statement since the 1987 election but opposition spokesperson Peter Shack has spoken in favour of privatization (Shack 1988), and the press has questioned whether health care is a right or a luxury (Editorial, *Canberra Times*, 25 May 1989: 8).

7 AA ACT CRS A1928, Item 195/13, Section 1; Item 500/1, Section 3; Item 700/1, Section 3; Item 690/39, Section 3; Item 690/13, Section 4

8 For a discussion of previous rulings on the extent of the federal spending power see Banting (1982: 52–4).

9 Conversation, Dr Alex Macpherson, 17 March 1987

10 Expansionism is not necessarily the same thing as policy innovation, of course. While social democrats often support expanded government activity, as they did in this case, they do no always do so. Problems of 'big' government such as unresponsiveness and delay have been criticized by writers from the length of the political spectrum. Further, terms such as 'innovative policy making,' 'reform government,' 'radical' policies, and so on, generally indicated the expansion of government activities, especially in social-policy areas until the mid-1970s. Since the collapse of the 'Keynesian-Collectivist Consensus,' these terms are increasingly likely to indicate an intention to reduce the size of government in general and of welfare programs in particular.

11 *Report of the Health Benefits Review* (1986: 38–9, 106–9); *Auckland Star*, 27 May 1987: A10

Bibliography

Abel-Smith, B. 1972. 'The History of Medical Care.' In E.W. Martin, ed., *Comparative Development of Social Welfare*, 219–40. London: George Allen and Unwin
– 1979. 'Foreword.' In Frank Honigsbaum, *The Division in British Medicine*, xiii–iv. London: Kogan Page
Abella, Irving. 1975. 'The Canadian Labour Movement, 1902–1960.' Historical Booklet no. 28. Ottawa: Canadian Historical Society
Acheson, R.M., and L. Aird, eds. 1976. *Seminars in Community Medicine*, vol. 1. London: Oxford University Press
Adie, Robert F., and Paul G. Thomas. 1982. *Canadian Public Administration*. Scarborough: Prentice-Hall
Advisory Council for Intergovernmental Relations. 1979a. *Intergovernmental Relations in the United States*, Information Paper no. 3. Canberra: AGPS
– 1979b. *Intergovernmental Relations in England*, Information Paper no. 4. Canberra: AGPS
– 1979c. *Relationship between Federal and State Governments in Australia*, Information Paper no. 6. Canberra: AGPS
– 1979d. *Relationships between Federal State and Local Governments*, Report 3. Canberra: AGPS
– 1980. *Federalism in West Germany*, Information Paper no. 8. Canberra: AGPS
– 1981a. *Local Government Systems of Australia*, Information Paper no. 7. Canberra: AGPS
– 1981b. *Towards Adaptive Federalism*, Information Paper no. 9. Canberra: AGPS
– 1982. *The Australian Loan Council and Intergovernmental Relations*, Report 5. Canberra: AGPS
Age Polls, 1975–86

Aitkin, Don. 1977. *Stability and Change in Australian Politics*. Canberra: Australian National University Press

Aldred, Jennifer, and John Wilkes, eds. 1983. *A Fractured Federation? Australia in the 1980's*. Sydney: George Allen and Unwin

Alford, Robert R. 1975. *Health Care Politics*. Chicago and London: University of Chicago Press

Andersen, Neville. 1984. 'Health Centres – An Overview.' *New Doctor* 34: 6–8

Anderson, Donald, and Anne Crichton. 1973. *What Price Group Practice?*, vols. 1 and 2. Distributed by the Office of the Coordinator Health Services Centre, University of British Columbia

Andreopoulos, S., ed. 1975. *National Health Insurance: Can We Learn from Canada?* Toronto: Wiley

Armitage, Andrew. 1975. *Social Welfare in Canada*. Toronto: McClelland and Stewart

Aucoin, Peter. 1974. 'Federal Health Care Policy.' In G. Bruce Doern and V. Seymour Wilson, eds., *Issues in Canadian Public Policy*, 55–84. Toronto: Macmillan of Canada

Auld, Douglas. 1979. 'Contemporary and Historical Economic Dimensions of Canadian Confederation,' *Occasional Paper no. 12*. Canberra: Centre for Research on Federal Financial Relations, Australian National University

Australian Archives ACT, Department of Health, Central Office, CA 17 CRS A1928, Correspondence Files, Multiple Number System, First Series

Australian Archives ACT, Department of Health, Central Office, CA 17 CRS A1658, Correspondence Files, Multiple Number System, Second Series

Australian Bureau of Statistics. 1987a. *Government Financial Estimates*, Catalogue no. 5501.0. Canberra: Government Printer

– 1987b. *Year Book: Australia 1986*. Canberra: Government Printer

Australian Community Health Association. 1986. *Review of the Community Health Program*. Sydney: Redfern Legal Centre Publishing

Australian Council of Social Services. 1973a. *Acoss Report on Accessibility of the Health Services*. Sydney

– 1973b. *A National Family Policy for Australia*, Discussion Paper

– 1978a. *Invest Now or Pay More Later*. Sydney

– 1978b. Medibank Bulletin I: *Bulk Billing*. Sydney

– 1978c. Medibank Bulletin II: *Deductibles*. Sydney

– 1981. *Share the Health*. Sydney

Australian Council of Trade Unions, Council of Government Employee Organisations. 1979. 'Budget Submissions: Background Information.' Typescript

– Peak Union Councils. 1980. 'Budget Submissions.' Typescript

– 1978a. *Health Care Costs Control Program*, Circular no. 151/1978

– 1978b. *Medibank Campaign*, Circular no. 171/1978

– 1981. *Information on Health Insurance Arrangements*, Social Welfare Research Unit
Australian Gallup Polls, 1941–70

Australian Institute of Health. 1986. *Australian Health Expenditures 1979–80 to 1981–82*. Canberra: AGPS

Australian Labor Party. 1902a. Federal Platform. *The Worker*, 13 December

– 1902b. Labor Platforms, State and Federal, Victoria

– 1902c. *Official Report of the Australian Labour Conference*, Sydney

– 1905. *Official Report of the Third Commonwealth Political Labour Conference*, Melbourne

– 1906. Labor Platforms, State and Federal, Victoria, *The Tocsin*, 21 June

– 1908. *Official Report of the Fourth Commonwealth Political Labour Conference*, Brisbane

– 1916. *Report of Proceedings of the Special Commonwealth Conference of the Australian Labor Party*, December, Melbourne

– 1919. *The Australian Labor Party's Message to the People of the Commonwealth*, General Elections, 13 December

– 1982. *The Hayden Health Plan*

– 1983. *Manifesto of the November Labor Conference*, New South Wales

– Early State and Federal Platforms held in the Petherick Room, Australian National Library

– *Federal Platforms* 1905, 1908, 1912, 1915, 1916, 1918, 1919, 1921, 1924, 1927, 1930, 1939, 1961, 1963, 1965, 1967, 1969, 1971, 1973, 1975, 1977, 1979, 1981, 1982, 1984

– *Official Reports of the Commonwealth Conference of the Australian Labor Party*, Fifth Conference 1912, Sixth Conference 1915, Seventh Conference 1918, Eighth Conference 1921, Tenth Conference 1924, Eleventh Conference 1927, Twelfth Conference 1930

Australian Medical Association. 1881–1914. *Australasian Medical Gazette*

– 1949. *A National Health Service*. Authorised by Dr J.G. Hunter, General Secretary, Federal Council of BMA in Australia

– 1969. *Paying for Health Care*. Glebe: Australian Medical Publishing Co.

– 1972. *Labor's Health Scheme*. Supplement to the AMA *Gazette*, 21 September

– 1972–86. *Annual Reports*

– 1973. AMA *Views on the Deeble Plan*. Glebe: Australasian Medical Publishing Co.

– 1989. *Medicover: Reform of Australia's Health Insurance System*, Green Paper, May. Sydney

– n.d. *Wran Attacks Doctors to Hide Govt. Waste*. New South Wales Branch, Sydney

– 3 February 1981, 19 February 1981, 29 April 1981. Press releases issued by Dr G. Repin, Secretary General

Australian Public Opinion Polls, 1970–86

Badgley, Robin F., and Samuel Wolfe. 1967. *Doctors' Strike*. Toronto: Macmillan of Canada

Banting, Keith. 1982. *The Welfare State and Canadian Federalism*. Montreal and Kingston: McGill-Queen's University Press

– 1985. 'Federalism and Income Security: Themes and Variations.' In T. Courchene et al, eds., *Ottawa and the Provinces: The Distribution of Money and Power,* 253–76. Toronto: Ontario Economic Council

– 1987. *The Welfare State and Canadian Federalism*, 2nd ed. Montreal and Kingston: McGill-Queen's University Press

– 1990. 'Social Policy in an Open Economy.' Paper presented to the Annual Meeting of the American Political Association, San Francisco, 30 August–2 September

Barer, Morris, and Robert Evans. 1989. 'Riding North on a Southbound Horse?' In Robert G. Evans and Greg L. Stoddart, eds. *Medicare at Maturity*, 53–163. Calgary: University of Calgary Press

Barnes, R.D., and R. Else-Mitchell. 1977. 'Aspects of the New Federalism Policy,' *Occasional Paper no. 7*. Canberra: Centre for Research on Federal Financial Relations, Australian National University

Bates, Erica. 1980. 'A Consumer's View of the Australian Experience in Health Insurance.' *The Lancet*, 5 July: 26–8

Battista, Renaldo, Robert Spasoff, and Walter Spitzer. 1989. 'Choice of Technique: Patterns of Medical Practices.' In G. Evans and Greg L. Stoddart, eds., *Medicare at Maturity*, 181–213. Calgary: University of Calgary Press

Bell, J. 1976. 'Queensland's Public Hospital System: Some Aspects of Finance and Control.' In J. Roe, ed., *Social Policy in Australia*. Stanmore: Cassell

Bella, Leslie. 1979. 'The Provincial Role in the Canadian Welfare State: The Influence of Provincial Social Policy Initiatives on the Design of the Canada Assistance Plan.' *Canadian Public Administration* 22(3): 438–52

Bellamy, David J., Tom H. Pammett, and Donald C. Rowat, eds. 1976. *Provincial Political Systems*. Toronto: Methuen

Better Health Commission. 1986a. *Interim Report*. Canberra: AGPS

– 1986b. *Final Report*, vols. 1–3. Canberra: AGPS

Birch A.H. 1955. *Federalism, Finance and Social Legislation*. Oxford: Clarendon Press

– 1975. 'Economic Models in Political Science: The Case of "Exit, Voice and Loyalty."' *British Journal of Political Science* 5(1): 59–82

Birman, John, ed. 1974. *The Health Problems of a Nation*. Perth: Extension Service, The University of Western Australia

Black, Edwin R. 1975. *Divided Loyalties: Canadian Concepts of Federalism*. Montreal and London: McGill University Press

Blaikie, the Hon. Bill. 1983. 'The Crisis of Medicare – An NDP View.' Typescript

Blake, Donald. 1982. 'The Consistency of Inconsistency: Party Identification in Federal and Provincial Politics.' *Canadian Journal of Political Science* 15(4): 691–710

Bland, F.A., ed. 1944. *Government in Australia*, 2nd ed. Sydney: Acting Government Printer

Blanpain, Jan. 1978. *National Health Insurance and Health Resources: The European Experience*. Cambridge, MA, and London, U.K.: Harvard University Press

Blewett, the Hon. Neal. 1983. Media Release, 22 July

– 1984. Media Release, 17 January

Blishen, Bernard R. 1969. *Doctors and Doctrines*. Toronto: University of Toronto Press

Boivin-Lesage, Monique. 1982. 'Quebec Marches towards State Medicine.' CMA *Journal* 127 (15 August): 314–15

Bolton, G.C. 1973. 'Louis Hartz,' *Australian Economic History Review* 12: 168–77

– 1974. '1939–51.' In F.K. Crowley, ed., *A New History of Australia*, 458–503. Melbourne: Heinemann

Bothwell, Robert, Ian Drummond, and John English. 1981. *Canada since 1945: Power, Politics, and Provincialism*. Toronto: University of Toronto Press

Brandis, George, Tom Harley, and Don Markwell, eds. 1984. *Liberals Face the Future*. Melbourne: Oxford University Press

Broadbent, the Hon. Edward. n.d. 'A New Employment Option for Canada.' Broadsheet

Brown, A.E. 1926. 'The Position of Public Hospitals in Relation to the Medical Profession.' *MJA* 9 October: 476–80

– 1951. 'The Development of Australian Hospitals in the Last Fifty Years.' *MJA* 6 January: 40–5

Brown, Malcolm. 1976. 'The Finance of Personal Health Services,' *Australian Quarterly* 48(3): 56–61

– 1977. *The Financing of Personal Health Services in New Zealand, Canada, and Australia*, Research Monograph no. 20. Canberra: Centre for Research on Federal Financial Relations, Australian National University

– 1983. *National Health Insurance in Canada and Australia*, Research Monograph no. 3. Canberra: Health Economics Research Unit, Australian National University

– 1984. *Established Program Financing: Evolution or Regression in Canadian Fiscal Federalism*, Research Monograph no. 38. Canberra: Centre for Research on Federal Financial Relations, Australian National University

Brunet, Jacques. 1981. 'An Overview of Developments in the Quebec Health Care System.' Paper presented at the 34th Annual Scientific Meeting of the

Gerontological Society of America and the 10th Annual Scientific and Educational Meeting of l'Association canadienne de gérontologie, Toronto, 8–12 November

Brunet, Jacques, et al. 1984. 'Health Priorities for Quebec: Scenario for the Year 2000.' Paper discussing the principal conclusions of the report on health promotion, Objectif: Santé. Typescript

Bryden, Kenneth. 1974. *Old Age Pensions and Policy Making in Canada.* Montreal and Kingston: McGill-Queen's University Press

Bunker, John. 1985. 'When Doctors Disagree.' *The New York Review* 25 April: 7–12

Butler, James, and Darrel Doessel, eds. 1986. *Economics and Health 1985.* Proceedings of the Seventh Australian Conference of Health Economists. Kensington: School of Health Administration, University of New South Wales

Byrne, Charles. 1943. *Proposal for the Future of Medical Practice.* Melbourne: Ramsay Ware

Cairns, Alan. 1977. 'The Government and Societies of Canadian Federalism.' *Canadian Journal of Political Science* 10(4): 495–725

– 1979. 'The Other Crisis in Canadian Federalism.' *Canadian Public Administration* 22: 175–95

Cameron, David R. 1978. 'The Expansion of the Public Economy: A Comparative Analysis.' *The American Political Science Review* 72: 1243–61

Canada. House of Commons. 1983–4. Bill C-3. 2nd Session, 32nd Parliament, 32–33 Elizabeth II

– *House of Commons Debates,* 1940–85

Canadian Health Coalition. 1983. Press Release, 14 December

– 1985. Open Letter to Members, Potential Members and Friends, Fall

Canadian Hospital Association. 1984. *Health Care Institutions in 1983: A Cross-Canada Overview.* Ottawa: Canadian Hospital Association

Canadian Medical Association. 1943. *The Medical Profession and Health Insurance.* A submission to the Special Committee on Social Security of the House of Commons. Pamphlet

– 1964. Report of the Special Committee to Adapt the Australian Health Plan to Canadian Conditions, Special Supplement, *CMA Journal* 91 (19 September)

– 1983. 'The Canada Health Act.' A Statement by Dr Everett L. Coffin, President. Typescript

Canadian Medical Association Journal. 1940–86

Canadian Nurses Association. 1983a. *Canada Health Act Bulletin,* 7 November

– 1983b. 'Canadian Nurses Say New Health Act Fails to Provide Needed Reforms.' Press Release, 12 December

Canaway, A.P. 1930. *The Failure of Federalism in Australia.* London: Oxford University Press

Careless, Anthony. 1984. 'The Struggle for Jurisdiction: Regionalism versus Rationalism.' *Publius* 14(1): 61–77

Carlson, Rick. 1985. 'Healthy People,' Supplement. *Canadian Journal of Public Health* 76 (May/June): 27–32

Carlton, the Hon. J.M. 1983a. 'Overview of Health Policy Dilemmas in Australia: The Federal Viewpoint.' Address at the Symposium, 'Dilemmas for Providers, Planners and Users of Health Services in Australia,' University of Sydney, 22 July

– 1983b. 'The Impact of Medicare.' Notes for address to Parramatta Special Branch of the Liberal Party, 25 July

– 1984. 'Official Launch – Opposition Health Policy.' Press Statement, 30 October

Carrigan, D. Owen. 1968. *Canadian Party Platforms*. Urbana: University of Illinois Press

Carter, George. 1980. 'New Directions in Financing Canadian Federalism,' *Occasional Paper no. 13*. Canberra: Centre for Research on Federal Financial Relations, Australian National University

Carty, R. Kenneth, and W. Peter Ward, eds. 1980. *Entering the Eighties: Canada in Crisis*. Toronto: Oxford University Press

Cassidy, Harry M. 1945. *Public Health and Welfare Reorganization*. Toronto: Ryerson Press

Castles, Francis G. 1978. *The Social Democratic Image of Society*. London: Routledge and Kegan Paul

– 1985. *The Working Class and Welfare*. Wellington: Allen and Unwin

– 1988. *Australian Public Policy and Economic Vulnerability*. Sydney: Allen and Unwin

– ed. 1982. *The Impact of Parties*. London: Sage

Castles, Frank, and Robert McKinlay. 1979a. 'Does Politics Matter: An Analysis of the Public Welfare Commitment in Advanced Democratic States.' *European Journal of Political Research* 7: 169–86

– 1979b. 'Public Welfare Provision, Scandinavia and the Sheer Futility of the Sociological Approach to Politics,' *British Journal of Political Science* 9(2): 157–71

Castonguay, Claude. 1975. 'The Quebec Experience: Effects on Accessibility.' In S. Andreopoulos, ed., *National Health Insurance: Can We Learn from Canada?*, 97–125. Toronto: Wiley

Chandler, William. 1977. 'Canadian Socialism and Policy Impact: Contagion from the Left?' *Canadian Journal of Political Science* 10(4): 755–80

Chesterman, Ester. 1986. 'Discussion.' In James Butler and Darrel Doessel, eds., *Economics and Health 1985*. Proceedings of the Seventh Australian Conference of Health Economists, 79–80. Kensington: School of Health Administration, University of New South Wales

Chorney, Harold, and Phillip Hanson. 1985. 'Neo-conservatism, Social Democracy and "Province-building": The Experience of Manitoba.' *Canadian Review of Sociology and Anthropology* 22(1): 1–29

Cilento, Sir Raphael. 1944. *Blueprint for the Health of a Nation.* Sydney: Scotow Press

Clague, Michael, Robert Dill, Roop Seebaran, and Brian Wharf. 1984. *Reforming Human Services.* Vancouver: University of British Columbia Press

CLSC Metro. 1983–4. *Annual Report.* Montreal

Coburn, David, Carl D'Arcy, Peter New, and George M. Torrance, eds. 1981. *Health and Canadian Society.* Toronto: Fitzhenry and Whiteside

Coffey, J. Edwin. 1984. 'Is Quebec Medicare Really a Model for Canada?' *CMA Journal* 130 (15 June): 1602–4

Cohen, Lynne. 1984. 'So You Want to Practise in British Columbia?' *CMA Journal* 130 (15 March): 793

Coleman, William D. 1984. *The Independence Movement in Quebec 1945–1980.* Toronto: University of Toronto Press

College of Physicians and Surgeons of Saskatchewan. 1960. Brief to the Advisory Planning Committee on Medical Care, December

Commonwealth Department of Health. 1966. *Guide to National Health Benefits.* Canberra

Commonwealth of Australia. 1900. Commonwealth of Australia Constitution Act, 63 and 64 Victoria, Chapter 12, 9 July

– 1973. *The Australian Health Insurance Plan,* White Paper. Canberra: AGPS

– 1979. *Progress in Health since 1976.* Canberra: Government Printer

– 1981. *Review of Commonwealth Functions.* Canberra: AGPS

– *Minutes of Proceedings.* Conferences of Commonwealth and State Ministers (Premiers' Conferences), January 1944, August 1944, 1947, 1948, 1949, 1950, 1951, 1953, 1955

– *Minutes of Proceedings.* Conferences of Ministers for Health for the Commonwealth and States of Australia, 1943, 1944, 1946, 1948, 1950, 1951

Commonwealth Parliamentary Debates, 1924–85

Community Health Association of NSW. 1981. *The Past, Present and Future of Community Health.* Sydney: NSW Community Health Association

Condliffe, J.B. 1959. *The Welfare State in New Zealand.* London: George Allen and Unwin

Contandriopoulos, Andre-Pierre, Claudine Laurier, and Louise-Helene Trottier. 1989. 'Towards an Improved Work Organization in the Health Services Sector: From Administrative Rationalization to Professional Rationality.' In Robert G. Evans and Greg L. Stoddart, eds., *Medicare at Maturity,* 287–328. Calgary: University of Calgary Press

Cooperative Commonwealth Federation. 1933. *Regina Manifesto, Programme of the Cooperative Commonwealth Federation adopted at First National Convention, July*

– 1956. *Winnipeg Declaration of the Principles of the Cooperative Commonwealth Federation.* New Democratic Party

Cooperative Health Centre, Prince Albert. 1980. Brief to the Hon. Emmett M. Hall, CCQC, Special Commissioner, Health Services Review, 1979

Courchene, Thomas. 1983. 'Canada's New Equalization Program: Description and Evaluation.' *Canadian Public Policy* 9(4): 458–75

Cranston, Ross. 1979. 'From Cooperative to Coercive Federalism and Back?' *Federal Law Review* 10: 121–42

Crisp, L.F 1949. *The Parliamentary Government of the Commonwealth of Australia.* London: Longmans Green

– n.d. *Ben Chifley.* London: Longmans

Crofts, Nick. 1985. 'Community Health: Where Do We Go From Here? – Preventive Interventions.' *New Doctor* 37: 9–11

Cumpston, Dr J.H.L. Commonwealth Director-General of Health. Papers, 1921–46. The Australian National Library, Canberra, ACT

Dampney, M. 1951. 'Health and Medical Services in Australia.' MA thesis, University of Melbourne

Daniels, John. 1984. 'The Recent NSW Dispute.' *New Doctor* 33: 3

Davies, A.F. 1964. *Australian Democracy,* 2nd ed. London: Longmans Green

Davis, G., J. Wanna, J. Warhurst, and P. Weller. 1988. *Public Policy in Australia.* Sydney: Allen and Unwin

Davis, R. 1987. 'The State of the States.' In Mark Birrell, ed., *The Australian States: Towards a Renaissance,* 18–37. Melbourne: Longman Cheshire

Davis, S. Rufus. 1951. 'Cooperative Federalism in Retrospect.' *Historical Studies* 5: 212–33

– 1955. 'The "Federal Principle" Reconsidered,' Parts 1 and 2. *Australian Journal of Politics and History* 1(1): 59–85; 1(2): 223–44

– 1978. *The Federal Principle: A Journey through Time in Quest of a Meaning.* Berkeley: University of California

Deber, R.B., and E. Vayda. 1985. 'The Environment of Health Policy Implementation: The Ontario, Canada Example.' In Walter Holland, Roger Detel, and George Knox, eds., *Oxford Textbook of Public Health,* vol. 3, 411–41. London: Oxford University Press

Deeble, J.S. 1970. 'Health Expenditures in Australia 1960–61 to 1966–67.' PhD thesis, University of Melbourne

– 1982a. 'Financing Health Care in a Static Economy.' *Social Science and Medicine* 16(6): 713–24

– 1982b. 'Unscrambling the Omelette: Public and Private Health Care Financing in Australia.' In G. McLachlan and A. Maynard, eds., *The Public/Private Mix in Health: The Myth and the Reality*, 425–63. London: Nuffield Provincial Hospitals Trust

Department of Finance. 1985. 'Fiscal Federalism in Canada: An Overview.' Typescript. Ottawa

Dewdney, J.C.H. 1972. *Australian Health Services*. Sydney: John Wiley

Diamond, Martin. 1963. 'What the Framers Meant by Federalism.' In Robert A. Goldwin, ed., *A Nation of States*, 24–41. Chicago: Rand McNally

– 1975. 'The Declaration and the Constitution: Liberty, Democracy and the Founders.' *The Public Interest* 41: 39–55

– 1977. *The Electoral College and the American Idea of Democracy*. Washington, DC: American Enterprise Institute for Public Policy Research

Dicey, A.V. 1959. *Introduction to the Study of the Law of the Constitution*, 10th ed. London: Macmillan

Dickey, Brian. 1976. 'The Labor Government and Medical Services in N.S.W., 1910–14.' In Jill Roe, ed., *Social Policy in Australia*, 60–73. Stanmore: Cassell Australia

– 1980a. *No Charity There*. Sydney: Nelson

– 1980b. 'The Politics of Hospital Finance: The Royal Prince Alfred Hospital, 1900–1914.' *Community Health Studies* 4(2): 111–20

Doern, G. Bruce, and Richard W. Phidd. 1983. *Canadian Public Policy*. Toronto: Methuen

Doern, G. Bruce, and V. Seymour Wilson, eds. 1974. *Issues in Canadian Public Policy*. Toronto: Macmillan of Canada

Donnison, David. 1976. 'An Approach to Social Policy.' *Australian Journal of Social Issues* 11(1): 4–31

Downs, Anthony. 1957. *An Economic Theory of Democracy*. New York: Harper and Brothers

– 1964. *Inside Bureaucracy*. Boston: Little Brown

Duckett, S.J. 1977. 'The Coordination of Services in Australia.' *Australian Journal of Social Issues* 12(3): 188–99

– 1979. 'Chopping and Changing Medibank,' Parts I and II. *Australian Journal of Social Issues* 14(3): 230–43; 15(2): 79–91

Duckett, S.J., and G.R. Palmer. 1981. 'Jamisonitis: A Case of Inadequate Diagnosis, Faulty Prescription and Uncertain Prognosis.' *New Doctor* 19: 10–14

Duncan, Graeme, ed. 1978. *Critical Essays in Australian Politics*. Melbourne: Edward Arnold

Duncan, W.G.K., ed. 1939. *Social Services in Australia*. Sydney: Angus and Robertson

Dundas, Colleen. 1984. 'Saskatchewan Physicians Bend on Extra–Billing.' CMA *Journal* 131 (15 December): 1947–84

Dussault, Rene. 1984. 'Professional Regulation in Canada: Effect on the Availability of Health Manpower.' In Robert G. Evans and Greg L. Stoddart, eds., *Medicare at Maturity*, 325–34. Calgary: University of Calgary Press

Dyck, Rand. 1976. 'The Canada Assistance Plan: The Ultimate in Cooperative Federalism.' *Canadian Public Administration* 19(4): 587–602

Dye, Thomas. 1966. *Politics, Economics and the Public: Public Policy Outcomes in the American States.* Chicago: Rand McNally

Eckstein, Harry. 1960. *Pressure Group Politics.* London: George Allen and Unwin

Edwards, John. 1976. 'The New Federalism?' *Current Affairs Bulletin* 53(5): 4–11

Elazar, D. 1962. *The American Partnership.* Chicago: University of Chicago Press

Elkins, David J., and Richard Simeon. 1980. *Small Worlds: Provinces and Parties in Canadian Political Life.* Toronto: Methuen

Elliott, Grant. 1984. 'The Division of Responsibility for Welfare in Australia.' *Australian Quarterly* 56(2): 172–82

Else-Mitchell R. 1975. 'The Rise and Demise of Coercive Federalism.' *Australian Journal of Public Administration* 36(2): 109–21

– 1979. 'Fiscal Equality between the States: The New Role of the Commonwealth Grants Commission.' *Australian Journal of Public Administration* 38(2): 157–67

– 1980. 'The Australian Federal Grants System and Its Impact on Fiscal Relations of the Federal Government with State and Local Governments.' *Australian Law Journal* 54: 480–8

– 1984. 'Fifty Years of the Commonwealth Grants Commission.' *Australian Journal of Public Administration* 43(3): 244–56

Elsten, the Hon. Murray. 1985. 'Remarks to the Public Information Forum, Ottawa, 26 October.' Typescript

Emy, Hugh V. 1978. *The Politics of Australian Democracy*, 2nd ed. Melbourne: Macmillan

Esman, Milton. 1984. 'Federalism and Modernisation: Canada and the United States.' *Publius* 14(1): 21–38

Evans, Gareth, ed. 1977. *Labor and the Constitution.* Melbourne: Heinemann

Evans, Robert. 1982. 'A Retrospective on the "New Perspective."' *Journal of Health Politics, Policy and Law* 7(2): 325–44

Everingham, Douglas. 1974. 'Health, a National Responsibility: The Labor Viewpoint.' In John Birnham, ed., *The Health Problems of a Nation*, 16–26. Perth: University of Western Australia

Feldman, Lionel, ed. 1981. *Politics and Government of Urban Canada*, 4th ed. Toronto: Methuen

Ferber, Helen. 1980. 'Diary of Legislative and Administrative Changes.' In R.B. Scotton and Helen Ferber, eds., *Public Expenditures and Social Policy in Australia*, Vol. 1. Melbourne: Longman Cheshire

Findlay, Peter. 1980. 'The Implications of "Sovereignty-Association" for Social Welfare Policy in Canada: An Anglophone Perspective.' *Canadian Journal of Social Work Education* 6 (Part I): 141–51

Fisher, the Hon. Andrew. 1909. Policy Speech, Gympie, Queensland, 30 March

Forbes, H.D. 1987. 'Hartz-Horowitz at Twenty: Nationalism, Toryism and Socialism in Canada and the United States.' *Canadian Journal of Political Science* 20(2): 386–419

Foulkes, R. 1973. *Health Security for British Columbians*, vol. 1. Victoria, BC: Health Security Programme Project

Fox, Paul W. 1982. 'Politics and Parties in Canada.' In Paul W. Fox, ed., *Politics: Canada*, 5th ed., 317–21. Toronto: McGraw-Hill Ryerson

Fraser, the Hon. Malcom. 1975. 'National Objectives – Social, Economic and Political Goals.' *Australian Quarterly* 47(1): 24–35

Freamo, B.E. 1982. 'How Hospitals Might Cope with Financial Restraint.' *CMA Journal* 127: 234–7

Freudenberg, Graham. 1977. *A Certain Grandeur*. Melbourne: Macmillan

Friedman, Milton, and Rose Friedman. 1980. *Free to Choose*. London: Penguin

Friedrich, C.J. 1968. *Trends of Federalism in Theory and Practice*. New York: Praeger

Fry, Denise. 1985. 'Health for All: Thinking Socially, Acting Locally.' *New Doctor* 37: 3–4

Fry, John A., ed. 1984. *Contradictions in Canadian Society*. Toronto: John Wiley

Fuchs, Victor. 1974. *Who Shall Live: Health, Economics and Social Policy*. New York: Basic Books

Fulcher, Derick. 1974. *Medical Care Systems*. Geneva: International Labour Office

Furler, Elizabeth. 1985. 'Women and Health: Radical Prevention.' *New Doctor* 37 (September): 5–8

Galligan, Brian. 1981. 'Federalism's Ideological Dimension and the Australian Labor Party.' *Australian Quarterly* 53(2): 128–40

– 1983. 'National Energy Policy in Canada and Australia.' *Australian-Canadian Studies: An Interdisciplinary Social Science Review* 1: 14–27

– 1984. 'Writing on Australian Federalism: The Current State of the Art.' *Australian Journal of Public Administration* 43(2): 177–86

Geekie, Douglas. 1982. 'CMA Must Prove the Health System Is Underfunded.' *CMA Journal* 126 (1 January): 77–8

– 1984. 'Ottawa Using the Health Stick to Tame Its Foes.' *CMA Journal* 120 (15 March): 754–5

Gelber, Sylvia M. 1980. 'The Path to Health Insurance.' In Carl A. Meilicke and

Janet L. Storch, eds., *Perspectives on Canadian Health and Social Services Policy: History and Emerging Trends,* 156–65. Ann Arbor, MI: Health Administration Press

Gibbins, Roger. 1982. *Territorial Politics in Canada and the United States.* Toronto: Butterworths

Glenday, Daniel, et al, eds. 1978. *Modernization and the Canadian State.* Toronto: Macmillan of Canada

Goldwin, Robert A. 1963. *A Nation of States.* Chicago: Rand McNally

Goode, Jim. 1981. 'The Road to Medibank Mark 10: Jamisonitis Revisited.' *New Doctor* 20: 10–12

Gosselin, Roger. 1984. 'Decentralisation/Regionalisation in Health Care: The Quebec Experience.' *HCM Review* Winter: 7–26

– 1985. 'The Quebec Health Care System in the Canadian Context: Impact on Medical Practice.' *Journal of Medical Practice Management* 1(1): 73–80

Government of Canada. 1927. Dominion-Provincial Conference, *Précis of Discussions.* Ottawa: Printer to the King's Most Excellent Majesty

– 1940. *Report of the Royal Commission on Dominion-Provincial Relations,* Books 1 and 2 (Rowell-Sirois Report). Ottawa: Printer to the King's Most Excellent Majesty

– 1943. *Report on Social Security for Canada* (Marsh Report). Ottawa: Printer to the King's Most Excellent Majesty

– 1946. Dominion-Provincial Conference, *Report of Proceedings.* Ottawa: Printer to the King's Most Excellent Majesty

– 1950. Federal-Provincial Conference, *Proceedings.* Ottawa: Printer to the King's Most Excellent Majesty

– 1955a. Federal-Provincial Conference, *Preliminary Meeting.* Ottawa: Queen's Printer

– 1955b. Federal-Provincial Conference, *Proceedings.* Ottawa: Queen's Printer

– 1957. Federal-Provincial Conference, *Proceedings.* Ottawa: Queen's Printer

– 1964. *Royal Commission on Health Services,* vol. 1 (Hall Report). Ottawa: Queen's Printer

– 1969. *Task Force Reports on the Cost of Health Services in Canada,* vols. 1–3. Ottawa

– 1973. *The Community Health Centre in Canada,* Report of the Community Health Centre Projects to the Ministries, vols. 1–3. Ottawa: Information Canada

– 1975. *The Federal Medical Care Program: Provincial Medical Care Insurance Plans.* Ottawa

– 1981a. *Federalism and Decentralization.* Ottawa: Minister of Supply and Services

– 1981b. *Report of the Parliamentary Task Force on Federal-Provincial Fiscal Arrangements* (Breau Report). Ottawa: Minister of Supply and Services

- 1982. *The Constitution Acts 1967–1982*. Ottawa: Department of Justice
- 1983a. 'Position Paper on Medicare.' News Release. Ottawa
- 1983b. *Preserving Universal Medicare*, White Paper. Ottawa
- 1985. *Privatization in the Canadian Health Care System: Assertions, Evidence, Ideology and Options*. Ottawa: Minister of Supply and Services
- Department of National Health and Welfare. 1984. *Basic Facts on Social Security Programs*. Ottawa
- Department of National Health and Welfare, 1985. Child and Elderly Benefits: Consultation Paper. Ottawa
Government of Manitoba. 1972. *White Paper on Health Policy*. Winnipeg: Department of Health and Social Development
Government of Ontario. 1974. *Report of the Health Planning Task Force* (Mustard Report). Toronto: Ministry of Health
Government of Quebec. 1970. *Report of the Commission of Inquiry on Health and Social Welfare* (Castonguay Report), vol. 4. Quebec City
- 1984. *Objectif: Santé*. Conseil des affaires sociales et de la famille
- 1985a. *Le Système de Santé et de Services Sociaux au Québec: Objectif: Santé*. Ministère des Affaires sociales
- 1985b. *Le Système de Santé et de Services Sociaux au Québec*: Annexe Statistique. Ministère des Affaires sociales
Granatstein, J.L. 1975. *Canada's War: The Politics of the Mackenzie King Government 1939–1945*. Toronto: Oxford University Press
Grant, C., and H.M. Lapsley. 1985. *The Australian Health Care System, 1984*, Australian Studies in Health Service Administration, no. 53. Kensington: University of New South Wales
Grant, Colin, and G.R. Palmer. 1975. 'Paying for Medical Care: The Methods in Other Countries.' *Current Affairs Bulletin* 51(8): 3–13
Gray, Gwen. 1982. 'The Termination of Medibank.' BA thesis, Australian National University, Canberra
- 1984. 'The Termination of Medibank.' *Politics* 19(2): 1–17
- 1987a. 'Health Policy in Two Federations.' PhD thesis, Australian National University, Canberra
- 1987b. 'Privatisation: An Attempt That Failed.' *Politics* 22(2): 15–28
- 1990. 'Health Policy and the Hawke Government: A Watershed?' In C. Jennett and R. Stewart, eds., *Consensus and Restructuring: Hawke and Australian Public Policy*, 223–44. Melbourne: Macmillan
- (forthcoming). 'Identifying the Differences: Policy Formulation in Canada and Australia – The Case of Legal Aid.' In B. Galligan and M. Alexander, eds., *Comparative Political Studies: Australia and Canada*. Melbourne: Longman Cheshire

Graycar, Adam, ed. 1978. *Perspectives in Australian Social Policy*. Melbourne: Macmillan
- 1979. *Welfare Politics in Australia*. Melbourne: Macmillan
- ed. 1983. *Retreat from the Welfare State*. Sydney: George Allen and Unwin
Green, David G., and Lawrence G. Cromwell. 1984. *Mutual Aid or Welfare State*. Sydney: George Allen and Unwin
Greenwood, G. 1946. *The Future of Australian Federalism*. Melbourne: Melbourne University Press
Grimes, the Hon. D. 1986. News Release, 4 December
Grodzins, Morton. 1967. 'The Federal System.' In A. Wildavsky, ed., *American Federalism in Perspective*, 109–43. Boston: Little Brown
Gross, Paul. 1977. 'Federalism Policy, Economic Policy and the Implementation of the Bailey Report.' *Australian Journal of Social Issues* 12(3): 201–7
Grossman, the Hon. Larry. 1982. 'Remarks to the Ontario Medical Association, Alliston Ontario, 16 October.' Typescript
Guest, Dennis. 1980a. 'A Response to Professor Findlay's Paper.' *Canadian Journal of Social Work Education* 6, Part 1: 152–5
- 1980b. *The Emergence of Social Security in Canada*. Vancouver: University of British Columbia Press
Gyarmati, Gabriel. 1975. 'The Doctrine of the Professions: Basis of a Power Structure.' *International Social Science Journal* 27(4): 629–53
Hall, E.M. 1980. *Canada's National-Provincial Health Program for the 1980's*. Health Services Review 1979. Saskatoon
Hamilton, Alexander, James Madison, and John Jay. 1961. *The Federalist*. Cambridge, MA: The Belknap Press of Harvard University
Hancock, Trevor. 1985. 'Beyond Health Care: From Public Health Policy to Healthy Public Policy.' Supplement 1, *Canadian Journal of Public Health* 76 (May/June): 9–11
Hardie, Miles. 1969. 'Islands of Change: A Review of Health Service Development in Britain.' *Hospital Administration* 14(3): 7–40
Hargrove, Erwin C. 1967. 'On Canadian and American Political Culture.' *Canadian Journal of Economics and Political Science* 33(1): 107–11
Hartz, Louis. 1964. *The Founding of New Societies: Studies in the History of the United States, Latin America, South Africa, Canada, and Australia*. New York: Harcourt, Brace and World
Harvey, Roy. 1981. 'Commentary: Unstated Assumptions, Partial Analysis and Unconscious Irony: The Jamison Report.' *Community Health Studies* 5(2): 156–71
Haskell, M.A. 1976. 'Decentralisation or Concentration of Power?' *Occasional Paper no. 3*. Canberra: Centre for Research on Federal Financial Relations, Australian National University

Hastings, J.E.F. 1978. 'Primary Health Care Services and Community Health Care Services.' *Canadian Journal of Public Health* 69: 95–7
– 1980. 'Federal-Provincial Insurance for Hospital and Physician's Care in Canada.' In Carl A. Meilicke and Janet L. Storch, eds., *Perspectives on Canadian Health and Social Services Policy: History and Emerging Trends*, 198–219. Ann Arbor, MI: Health Administration Press
Hastings, J.E.F., and W. Mosley. 1980. 'Introduction: The Evolution of Organized Community Health Services in Canada.' In Carl A. Meilicke and Janet L. Storch, eds., *Perspectives on Canadian Health and Social Services Policy: History and Emerging Trends*, 145–55. Ann Arbor, MI: Health Administration Press
Hastings, John E.F., and Eugene Vayda. 1989. 'Health Services Organization and Delivery: Promise and Reality.' In Robert G. Evans and Greg L. Stoddart, eds., *Medicare at Maturity*, 198–219. Calgary: University of Calgary Press
Hawker, Geoffrey, R.F.I. Smith, and Patrick Weller. 1979. *Politics and Policy in Australia.* St Lucia: University of Queensland Press
Hayden, Bill. 1974. 'Planning and Integration of Welfare Services: An Australian Government Viewpoint.' *Australia Journal of Social Issues* 9(1): 3–10
Hayden, Hon. W.G., Minister for Social Security. Files, 1972–5
Hayek, F.H. 1949. *Individualism and the Economic Order.* London: Routledge and Kegan Paul
Hazelhurst, Cameron, ed. 1979. *Australian Conservatism.* Canberra: Australian National University Press
Heagerty, J.J. 1980. 'The Development of Public Health in Canada.' In Carl A. Meilicke and Janet L. Storch, eds., *Perspectives on Canadian Health and Social Services Policy: History and Emerging Trends*, 137–44. Ann Arbor, MI: Health Administration Press
Health Benefits Review. 1986. *Choices for Health Care*, Report of the Health Benefits Review. Wellington, NZ: Government Printer
Health Care Providers. 1981. Press Release, 29 January
Health Insurance Commission. 1975–85. *Annual Reports.* Canberra: AGPS
Health Issues Centre. 1986. *Health Issues*, November/December
– 1987. *Medicare: A Double-Edged Sword.* February
Heclo, Hugh. 1972. 'Review Article: Policy Analysis.' *British Journal of Political Science* 2(1): 83–108
– 1974. *Modern Social Politics in Britain and Sweden.* New Haven: Yale University Press
Heidenheimer, Arnold J., Hugh Heclo, and Carolyn Teich Adams. 1983. *Comparative Public Policy*, 2nd ed. London: Macmillan
Heller, Francis. 1981. 'Is There a Theory of Federalism?' *Political Science Reviewer* 11: 287–310

Henderson, Ronald F., ed. 1981. *The Welfare Stakes*. Melbourne: Institute of Applied Economic and Social Research

Hicks, Neville, and Jan Powning. 1983. 'Commentary: Preparing for the Second Community Health Program.' *Community Health Studies* 7(3): 320–8

Higgins, Donald. 1977. *Urban Canada: Its Government and Politics*. Toronto: Macmillan of Canada

Hill, Michael, and Glen Bramley. 1986. *Analysing Social Policy*. Oxford: Basil Blackwell

Hirst, J.B. 1984. 'Keeping Colonial History Colonial: The Hartz Thesis Revisited.' *Historical Studies* 21(82): 85–104

Hockin, T.A. 1976. *Government in Canada*. Toronto: McGraw-Hill Ryerson

Hodgins, Bruce W. 1978. 'The Plans of Mice and Men.' In Bruce W. Hodgins, Bruce, Don Wright, and W.H. Heick, eds., *Federalism in Canada and Australia: The Early Years*, 3–18. Canberra: Australian National University Press

Hodgins, Bruce W., and Don Wright. 1978. 'Canada and Australia: Continuing but Changing Federations.' In Bruce W. Hodgins, Don Wright, and W.H. Heick, eds., *Federalism in Canada and Australia: The Early Years*, 289–304. Canberra: Australian National University Press

Hogg, Peter W. 1985. *Constitutional Law of Canada*. Toronto: Carswell

Hollborn, Joan. 1962. 'Bungle, Truce and Trouble.' Booklet reprinted from a series of articles by the author published in the *Globe and Mail*, December

Holmes, Jean, and Campbell Sharman. 1977. *The Australian Federal System*. Sydney: George Allen and Unwin

Honigsbaum, Frank. 1979. *The Division in British Medicine*. London: Kogan Page

Horn, Michiel. 1980. *The League for Social Reconstruction: Intellectual Origins of the Democratic Left in Canada 1930–42*. Toronto: University of Toronto Press

– 1984. *The Great Depression of the 1930's in Canada*, Historical Booklet no. 39. Ottawa: Canadian Historical Association

Horowitz, G. 1966. 'Conservatism, Liberalism and Socialism in Canada: An Interpretation.' *Canadian Journal of Economics and Political Science* 32(2): 145–71

Hospitals and Health Services Commission. 1976. *Review of the Community Health Program*. Canberra: AGPS

– 1978. *A Discussion Paper on Paying for Health Care*. Canberra: AGPS

Hospitals and Health Services Commission, Interim Committee. 1973. *Report on a Community Health Program for Australia*. Canberra: AGPS

Hum, Derek. 1983. *Federalism and the Poor: A Review of the Canada Assistance Plan*. Ontario Economic Council

Hunter, Thelma. 1963. 'Some Thoughts on the Pharmaceutical Benefits Scheme.' *Australian Journal of Social Issues* 1(4): 32–42

– 1965. 'Pharmaceutical Benefits Legislation, 1944–50.' *Economic Record* 41: 412–25

- 1966. 'Planning Health Policy in Australia, 1941–45.' *Public Administration* 44: 315–32
- 1968. 'The Politics of National Health.' PhD thesis, Australian National University, Canberra
- 1980. 'Pressure Groups and the Australian Political Process: The Case of the Australian Medical Association.' *Journal of Commonwealth and Comparative Politics* 18(2): 190–206

Illich, Ivan. 1975. *Medical Nemesis: The Expropriation of Health.* London: Marion Boyars

Inglis, K.S. 1958. *Hospital and Community.* Melbourne: Melbourne University Press

Ismail, Jacqueline S., ed. 1985. *Canadian Social Welfare Policy.* Montreal and Kingston: McGill-Queen's University Press

Jaensch, Dean. 1977. *The Politics of 'New Federalism.'* Adelaide: Australian Political Studies Association
- 1983. *The Australian Party System.* Sydney: George Allen and Unwin

Jenkins, Shirley, ed. 1969. *Social Security in International Perspective.* New York: Columbia University Press

Joint Committee on Social Security. 1943. *Sixth Interim Report.* Canberra: Government Printer
- 1944. *Seventh Interim Report.* Canberra: Government Printer
- 1945. *Eighth Interim Report.* Canberra: Government Printer

Jones, Elwood H. 1978. 'Localism and Federalism in Upper Canada to 1865.' In Bruce W. Hodgins, Don Wright, and W.H. Heick, eds., *Federalism in Canada and Australia: The Early Years,* 19–42. Canberra: Australian National University Press

Jupp, James. 1982. *Party Politics: Australia 1966–81.* North Sydney: George Allen and Unwin

Katzenstein, Peter. 1985. *Small States in World Markets.* Ithaca: Cornell University Press

Kay, Barry J. 1977. 'An Examination of Class and Left-Right Party Images in Canadian Voting.' *Canadian Journal of Political Science* 10(1): 127–43

Kellow, A. 1981. 'Political Science and Political Theory.' *Politics* 16(1): 33–45
- 1988. 'Australian Federalism: The Need for New Zealand (as well as Canadian) Comparisons.' *Australian-Canadian Studies* 6(1): 59–72

Kewley, T.H. 1973. *Social Security in Australia 1900–72,* 2nd ed. Sydney: Sydney University Press

Key, V.O. 1952. *Politics, Parties and Pressure Groups,* 3rd ed. New York: Thomas Y. Crowell
- 1961. *Public Opinion and American Democracy.* New York: Alfred A. Knopf

King, Anthony. 1973. 'Ideas, Institutions and the Policies of Government.' *British Journal of Political Science* 3(3): 291–314; 3(4): 409–24

Klein, Rudolf. 1971. 'Accountability in the National Service.' *Political Quarterly* 42: 363–75

– 1974. 'The Case for Elitism: Public Opinion and Public Policy.' *Political Quarterly* 45(4): 406–17

– 1976. 'Political Models and the National Health Service.' In Roy M. Acheson and Leslie Aird, eds., *Seminars in Community Medicine*, vol. 1. London: Oxford University Press

– 1977. 'The Corporate State, the Health Service and the Professions.' *New University Quarterly* 31(2): 160–80

Korcok, Milan. 1982. 'Underfunding's Effect on Canadian Hospitals.' CMA *Journal* 127 (1 September): 409–13

Lalonde, M. 1974. *A New Perspective on the Health of Canadians*. Ottawa: Information Canada

Lane, W.R. 1975. 'Financial Relations and Section 96.' *Public Administration* 34(1): 45–72

Lapierre, Laurier, J. McLeod, C. Taylor, and W. Young, eds. 1971. *Essays on the Left*. Toronto: McClelland and Stewart

Larkin, John. 1989. 'The New South Wales Doctors' Dispute 1984–85 – An Interpretation.' *Politics* 24(2): 67–78

Larson, Magali. 1979. 'Professionalism: Rise and Fall.' *International Journal of Health Services* 9(4): 607–27

Laski, Harold. 1939. 'The Obsolescence of Federalism.' *New Republic* 3 May: 307–9

Le Grand, J. 1982. *The Strategy of Equality*. London: George Allen and Unwin

Leach, Richard. 1984. 'Canadian Federalism Revisited.' *Publius* 14(1): 9–19

Leach, S., and John Stewart, eds. 1982. *Approaches in Public Policy*. Sydney: Institute of Local Government Studies, George Allen and Unwin

Lee, Sidney S. 1979. *Quebec's Health System: A Decade of Change, 1967–1977,* Monograph no. 4. The Institute of Public Administration of Canada

Leggett, C.A.C. 1976. 'Organisation and Development of Queensland Hospitals in the Twentieth Century.' MA thesis, University of Queensland

Leman, Christopher. 1977. 'Patterns of Policy Development: Social Security in the United States and Canada.' *Public Policy* 25(2): 261–91

Lennie, Ian, and Alan Owen. 1983. 'Continuing Crisis in Health Services.' *Community Health Studies* 7(3): 227–37

Leslie, Peter M. 1987. *Federal State, National Economy*. Toronto: University of Toronto Press

Liberal Party of Australia. 1948, 1960, 1974, 1982. Federal Platforms of the Liberal Party of Australia

- 1949. *The Liberal Way of Progress*. Sydney: Liberal Party of Australia
- 1964. *We Believe*. A statement of Liberal Party beliefs. 9th reprint. Canberra: Liberal Party of Australia
- 1969. *Policy Speech*. Prime Minister John Gorton, plus Supplementary Statement on Health. Canberra: Liberal Party of Australia
- 1972. *National Health Policies*, A Liberal Party Publication
- 1974. *The Way Ahead with a Liberal–Country Party Government*. Health and Social Security Policy
- 1975a. *Federalism Policy*. Canberra: Paragon Printers
- 1975b. *The New Government Policies*
- 1978. *Federalism and the Liberal Philosophy*
- 1983a. *Liberal – Moving Ahead*, 36th Federal Council
- 1983b. 'We're Not Waiting for the World.' Policy Speech, Prime Minister Malcolm Fraser
- 1983c. *Facing the Facts* (Valder Report). Report of the Liberal Party Committee of Review
- 1984. 'Policy on Health.' Typescript
Liberal Party of Canada. 1982. *Liberal Policy Newletter*. Autumn
- 1982. *Report on 1980 Resolutions to the National Convention*, Ottawa, November
- 1982–3. *Liberal Policy Newsletter*. Winter
- 1983. *Report to the Standing Committee on Policy on Action Taken on the 1982 National Convention Resolutions*
- 1984. '1984 Briefing Book.' Typescript
Lijphart, Arend. 1971. 'Comparative Politics and Comparative Method.' *The American Political Science Review* 65: 682–93
Lipset, S.M. 1950. *Agrarian Socialism*. Berkeley: University of California Press
Livingston, William S. 1967. 'A Note on the Nature of Federalism.' In Aaron Wildavsky, ed., *American Federalism in Perspective*, 33–47. Boston: Little Brown
Lockhart-Gibson, J. 1909. 'Hospital Abuse.' *The Australian Medical Gazette* 20 January: 15–18
Lomas, Jonathon. 1985. *First and Foremost in Community Health Centres*. Toronto: University of Toronto Press
Lovell-Smith, J.B. 1966. *The New Zealand Doctor and the Welfare State*. Auckland: Blackwood and Janet Paul
Lower, A.R.M., and F.R. Scott. 1958. *Evolving Canadian Federalism*. Durham: Duke University Press
Lowi, Theodore J. 1964. 'American Business, Public Policy, Case Studies and Political Theory.' *World Politics* 16: 677–715
- 1984. 'Why Is There No Socialism in the United States? A Federal Analysis.' *International Political Science Review* 5(4): 369–80

Lyons, the Hon. J.A. 1931. Policy Speech, Sydney, 2 December

Macpherson, Ian. 1979. *The Cooperative Movement on the Prairies 1900–1955*. Canadian Historical Association Booklet No. 33. Ottawa: The Canadian Historical Association

Maddox, Graham. 1973. 'Federalism: Or Government Frustrated.' *Australian Quarterly* 56(3): 92–100

Madison, James. 1961. In Alexander Hamilton, James Madison, and John Jay, *The Federalist*. Cambridge: The Belknap Press of Harvard University

Magnusson, Warren, W.K. Carroll, C. Doyle, M. Langer, and R.B.J. Walker, eds. 1984. *The New Reality*. Vancouver: New Star Books

Mallory, J.R. 1954. *Social Credit and the Federal Power in Canada*. Toronto: University of Toronto Press

– 1977. 'The Five Faces of Federalism.' In J. Peter Meekison, ed., *Canadian Federalism: Myth or Reality*, 3rd ed., 19–30. Toronto: Methuen

Manga, Pranal, and Geoffrey Weller. 1980. 'The Failure of the Equity Objective in Health: A Comparative Analysis of Canada, Britain and the United States.' *Comparative Social Research* 3: 229–67

Manne, Robert, ed. 1982. *The New Conservatism in Australia*. Melbourne: Oxford University Press

Marmor, Theodore R. 1983. *Political Analysis and American Medical Care*. Cambridge: Cambridge University Press

Marmor, Theodore R., and David Thomas. 1972. 'Doctors, Politics and Pay Disputes: "Pressure Group Politics" Revisited.' *British Journal of Political Science* 2(4): 421–42

Martin, A.W. 1982. 'Australian Federalism and Nationalism: Historical Notes.' In R.L. Mathews, ed., *Public Policies in Two Federal Countries: Canada and Australia*, 27–46. Canberra: Centre for Research on Federal Financial Relations, Australian National University

Mathews, R.L., ed. 1974. *Intergovernmental Relations in Australia*. Sydney: Angus and Robertson

– ed. 1976. *Making Federalism Work*. Canberra: Australian National University Press

– 1979. *Australian Federalism 1978*. Canberra: Centre for Research on Federal Financial Relations, Australian National University

– 1980. *Australian Federalism 1979*. Canberra: Centre for Research on Federal Financial Relations, Australian National University

– ed. 1982. *Public Policies in Two Federal Countries: Australia and Canada*. Canberra: Centre for Research on Federal Financial Relations, Australian National University

– 1983. 'The Commonwealth-State Financial Contract.' In Jennifer Aldred and

John Wilkes, eds., *A Fractured Federation? Australia in the 1980's*. Sydney: George Allen and Unwin

Mathews, R.L., and W.R.C. Jay. 1972. *Federal Finance*. Melbourne: Nelson

Mathews, R.L., R.H. Scott, P. deLacy, and C. Saunders. 1982. *Australian Federalism 1980*. Canberra: Centre for Research on Federal Financial Relations, Australian National University

Mathews, Russell. 1976. 'The Changing Pattern of Australian Federalism,' *Reprint Series no. 17*. Canberra: Centre for Research on Federal Financial Relations, Australian National University

– 1977. 'Philosophical, Political and Economic Conflicts in Australian Federalism,' *Reprint Series no. 23*. Canberra: Centre for Research on Federal Financial Relations, Australian National University

– 1978. *Australian Federalism 1977*. Canberra: Centre for Research on Federal Financial Relations, Australian National University

Matthews, Trevor. 1976. 'Australian Pressure Groups.' In Henry Mayer and Helen Nelson, eds., *Australian Politics: A Reader*. Melbourne: Cheshire

Maxwell, James. 1974. 'Federal Grants in Canada, Australia and the United States.' *Publius* 2(4): 63–75

May, Ronald. 1970. 'Decision-Making and Stability in Federal Systems.' *Canadian Journal of Political Science* 3(1): 73–87

Mayer, Henry. 1956. 'Some Conceptions of the Australian Party System 1910–1950.' *Historical Studies* 7(27): 253–70

– ed. 1973. *Australia's Political Pattern*. Melbourne: Longman Cheshire

Maynard, Alan. 1975. *Health Care in the European Community*. London: Croom Helm

McCarty, J.W. 1973. 'Australia as a Region of Recent Settlement in the Nineteenth Century.' *Australian Economic History Review* 12: 148–67

McEwan, E. Duncan. 1979. 'Whatever Happened to the Lalonde Report?' *Canadian Journal of Public Health* 70: 13–16

McGrath, A.G. 1975. 'The History of Medical Organisation in Australia.' PhD thesis, University of Sydney

McKeown, Thomas. 1976a. *The Modern Rise of Population*. London: Edward Arnold

– 1976b. *The Role of Medicine*. London: Nuffield Provincial Hospitals Trust

McLachlan, Gordon, and Alan Maynard, eds. 1982. *The Public/Private Mix for Health*. London: Nuffield Provincial Hospitals Trust

McLarty, R.A. 1980a. 'Current Issues in Canadian Fiscal Federalism,' *Reprint Series, no. 36*. Canberra: Centre for Research on Federal Financial Relations, Australian National University

– 1980b. 'Federalism in Canada and Australia: Where Might We Go from Here?'

Reprint Series no. 35. Canberra: Centre for Research on Federal Financial Relations, Australian National University

McLeod, Jack. 1971. 'Health, Wealth, and Politics.' In Laurier Lapierre et al., eds., *Essays on the Left*, 81–99. Toronto: McClelland and Stewart

McLeod, John T. 1982. 'Explanations of Our Party System.' In Paul W. Fox, ed., *Politics: Canada*, 5th ed., 310–16. Toronto: McGraw-Hill Ryerson

McMillan, John, Gareth Evans, and Haddon Storey. 1983. *Australia's Constitution: Time for Change?* Sydney: Law Foundation of New South Wales and George Allen and Unwin

McMinn, W.G. 1979. *A Constitutional History of Australia.* Melbourne: Oxford University Press

Mechanic, David. 1979. *Future Issues in Health Care.* New York: The Free Press

Medical Journal of Australia, 1915–86

Meekison, J. Peter, ed. 1977. *Canadian Federalism: Myth or Reality,* 3rd ed. Toronto: Methuen

Meilicke, Carl A., and Janet L. Storch, eds. 1980. *Perspectives on Canadian Health and Social Policy: History and Emerging Trends.* Ann Arbor, MI: Health Administration Press

Meisel, John. 1960. 'The Formulation of Liberal and Conservative Programmes in the 1957 Canadian General Election.' *Canadian Journal of Economics and Political Science* 36(4): 565–74

Mendelsohn, Ronald. 1965. 'The Introduction of the Commonwealth-State Tuberculosis Scheme 1948–1952.' In B.B. Schaffer and D.C. Corbett, eds., *Decisions: Case Studies in Australian Administration,* 104–23. Melbourne: F.W. Cheshire

– ed. 1982. *Social Welfare Finance: Selected Papers.* Canberra: Centre for Research on Federal Financial Relations, Australian National University

– ed. 1983. *Australian Social Welfare Finance.* Canberra: George Allen and Unwin in Association with the Centre for Research on Federal Financial Relations, Australian National University

Menzies, Sir Robert. 1967. *Central Power in the Australian Commonwealth.* Charlottesville: University Press of Virginia

Mercer, William M. 1986. *International Benefits Guidelines 1986.* London: N.M. Mercer International

Metcalfe, A.J. 1951. 'The Growth and Development of Public Health Services in Australia During Fifty Years.' *MJA* 6 January: 45–51

Milio, Nancy. 1981. 'Promoting Health through Structural Change: Analysis of the Origins and Implementation of Norway's Farm-Food–Nutrition Policy.' *Social Science and Medicine* 15: 721–34

– 1983. 'Commentary: Next Steps in Community Health Policy: Matching Rhetoric with Reality.' *Community Health Studies* 7(2): 185–92

Milner, Henry. 1984. 'Who Really Won When Quebec Voted "No"?' In John A. Fry, ed., *Contradictions in Canadian Society*, 265–75. Toronto: John Wiley

Mishra, Ramesh. 1984. *The Welfare State in Crisis*. Brighton: Wheatsheaf Books

Monsen, R. Joseph, and Anthony Downs. 1971. 'Public Goods and Private Status.' *Public Interest* 23: 64–76

Moodie, Graeme C., and Gerald Studdert-Kennedy. 1970. *Opinions, Publics and Pressure Groups*. London: George Allen and Unwin

Morgan Gallup Polls, 1975–85

Morley, J.B., R.G. Taylor, and L.J. Opit. 1982. 'Patterns of Private Hospital Ownership in Victoria.' *Community Health Studies* 6(1): 25–9

Morreale, Joseph. 1981. 'Is National Health Insurance the Best We Can Do?' *Health Policy Quarterly* 1(2): 125–41

Moscovitch, Allan. 1983. *The Welfare States in Canada*. Waterloo: Wilfrid Laurier University Press

Moulton-Barrett, Donalee. 1985. 'Nova Scotia: Risking Rights to the Political Process.' *CMA Journal* 132 (1 February): 279–80

Moyes, E.A. 1984. 'A Critical Analysis of the Canada Health Act and Its Impact on the Administration of Health Care in British Columbia.' Master of Public Administration thesis, University of Victoria

Nathan, Richard. 1975. 'The New Federalism versus the Emerging New Structuralism.' *Publius* 5(3): 111–29

National Council of Welfare. 1978. *The Refundable Child Tax Credit*. Ottawa

– 1979. *Women and Poverty*. Ottawa

– 1981. Submission to the Parliamentary Task Force on Federal–Provincial Fiscal Arrangements. Ottawa

– 1982a. 'The June 1982 Budget and Social Policy.' Typescript

– 1982b. *Medicare: The Public Good and Private Practice*. Ottawa: Minister of Supply and Services

– 1984. *1984 Poverty Lines*. Ottawa: Minister of Supply and Services

– 1985a. *Giving and Taking: The 1985 Budget and the Poor*. Ottawa: Minister of Supply and Services

– 1985b. *Opportunity for Reform*. Ottawa: Minister for Supply and Services

National Insurance Commission. 1938. *National Insurance: A Summary of the Principles of the Australian National Health and Pensions Insurance Act 1938*. Canberra: Government Printer

Naylor, C.D. 1982. 'In Defense of Medicare.' *Canadian Forum* April: 12–16

– 1986. *Private Practice, Public Payment*. Montreal and Kingston: McGill-Queen's University Press

Naylor, David, and Adam L. Linton. 1986. 'Allocation of Health Care Resources: A Challenge for the Medical Profession.' *CMA Journal* 134 (15 February): 333–40

Neumann, Franz. 1957. *The Democratic and the Authoritorian State.* Glencoe, IL: The Free Press

New Democratic Party. 1976. *New Democratic Politics 1961–1976.* Ottawa: Mutual Press

- 1977. *Convention Resolutions 1977.* Ottawa: New Democratic Party
- 1979. *Convention Resolutions 1979.* Ottawa: New Democratic Party
- 1981. *Convention Resolutions 1981.* Ottawa: New Democratic Party
- 1983a. *No Cause for Rejoicing,* Task Force on Older Women in Canada. Ottawa: New Democratic Party of Canada and Participation of Women Committee
- 1983b. *Women's Policy Manual.* Ottawa: New Democratic Party
- 1985a. *Convention 85,* Constitution of the New Democratic Party
- 1985b. *Convention 85, Resolutions Passed,* 13th Federal NDP Convention, Ottawa, July 1985
- n.d. *A Place for Crown Corporations.* No. 8 of a series produced by the Educational Materials Committee, Office of Lynn McDonald, MP for Broadview–Greenwood
- n.d. *Dialogue with Voters.* No. 13 of a series produced by the Educational Materials Committee, Office of Lynn McDonald, MP for Broadview–Greenwood
- n.d. *How Much Government?* No. 9 of a series produced by the Educational Materials Committee, Office of Lynn McDonald, MP for Broadview–Greenwood
- n.d. *Medicare – Canada's Pride.* No. 11 of a series produced by the Educational Materials Committee, Office of Lynn McDonald, MP for Broadview–Greenwood
- n.d. *Multiculturalism and the NDP.* No. 12 of a series produced by the Educational Materials Committee, Office of Lynn McDonald, MP for Broadview–Greenwood
- n.d. *New Democrats and Balanced Budgets.* No. 5 of a series produced by the Educational Materials Committee, Office of Lynn McDonald, MP for Broadview–Greenwood
- n.d. *Reaganomics and Thatcherism.* No. 3 of a series produced by the Educational Materials Committee, Office of Lynn McDonald, MP for Broadview–Greenwood
- n.d. *Restraint – B.C. Style.* No. 6 of a series produced by the Educational Materials Committee, Office of Lynn McDonald, MP for Broadview–Greenwood
- n.d. *Social Democracy.* No. 1 of a series produced by the Educational Materials Committee, Office of Lynn McDonald, MP for Broadview–Greenwood
- n.d. *Stewardship of Our Resources.* No. 10 of a series produced by the Educational Materials Committee, Office of Lynn McDonald, MP for Broadview–Greenwood

- n.d. *The Social Gospel.* No. 2 of a series produced by the Educational Materials Committee, Office of Lynn McDonald, MP for Broadview–Greenwood
- n.d. *Unemployment: Who Profits?* No. 4 of a series produced by the Educational Materials Committee, Office of Lynn McDonald, MP for Broadview–Greenwood
- n.d. *What about Inflation?* No. 7 of a series produced by the Educational Materials Committee, Office of Lynn McDonald, MP for Broadview–Greenwood

Newman, Morris J. 1924. 'National Insurance in Australia as Affecting the Medical Profession.' *MJA* 8 March: 227–34

Niskanen, William A. 1971. *Bureaucracy and Representative Government.* Chicago: Aldine

NSW Department of Health. 1986. *Area Health Services,* State Health Publication no. 86–066. Sydney

OECD. 1985. *Measuring Health Care 1960–1983.* Paris
- 1987. *Revenue Statistics (1965–1986).* Paris

Ogilvie, A.G. 1938. 'State Medical Services in Tasmania.' *Australian Quarterly* 10(3): 57–64

Oliver, Michael, ed. 1961. *Social Purpose for Canada.* Toronto: University of Toronto Press

Olson, Mancur. 1965. *The Logic of Collective Action.* Cambridge: Harvard University Press

Ontario Economic Council. 1976. *Ontario Economic Council, Issues and Alternatives 1976: Health.* Toronto

Opit, L.J. 1983. 'Wheeling, Healing and Dealing: The Political Economy of Health Care in Australia.' *Community Health Studies* 7(3): 238–46

Ostrom, V. 1969. 'Operational Federalism: Organisation for the Provision of Public Services in the American Federal System.' *Public Choice* 6: 1–17
- 1973. 'Can Federation Make a Difference?' *Publius* 3(2): 197–237
- 1987. *The Political Theory of the Compound Republic: Designing the American Experiment,* 2nd ed. Lincoln: University of Nebraska Press

Page, Sir Earle. 1963. *Truant Surgeon.* Sydney: Angus and Robertson
- Papers. The Australian National Library, Canberra, ACT, MS 1633

Palmer, G.R. 1978. 'Cost Escalation and Cost Containment in the Australian Health Services.' *Current Affairs Bulletin* 55(5): 15–23

Panitch, Leo, ed. 1977. *The Canadian Economy and Political Power.* Toronto: University of Toronto Press

Parker, Robert. 1973. 'Federalism – Australian Brand.' In H. Mayer, ed., *Australia's Political Pattern,* 254–63. Melbourne: Longman Cheshire

Parliament of the Commonwealth of Australia. 1969. *Report from the Senate Select*

Committee on Medical and Hospital Costs. Canberra: Commonwealth Government Printing Office

Parsons, Arthur. 1985. 'Allocating Health Care Resources: A Moral Dilemma.' *CMA Journal* 132 (15 February): 466–9

Patience, Allan, and Brian Head, eds. 1979. *From Whitlam to Fraser.* Melbourne: Oxford University Press

Patience, Allan, and Jeffrey Scott, eds. 1983. *Australian Federalism: Future Tense.* Melbourne: Oxford University Press

Paul, J.B. 1979. 'Australian Federalism.' In Richard Lucy, ed., *The Pieces of Politics,* 2nd ed., 258–78. Melbourne: Macmillan

Pensabene, T.S. 1980. *The Rise of the Medical Profession in Victoria,* Research Monograph 2. Canberra: Health Research Project, Australian National University

– 1986. 'Implications of the New South Wales Doctor's Dispute.' In James Butler and Darrel Doessel, eds., *Economics and Health 1985.* Proceedings of the Seventh Australian Conference of Health Economists, 67–78. Kensington: School of Health Administration, University of New South Wales

Phillips, P.D. 1965. 'Federalism and the Provision of Social Services.' In Keith Hancock, ed., *The National Income and Social Welfare,* 39–60. Melbourne: Cheshire

Pineault, Raynald. 1984. 'The Place of Prevention in the Quebec Health Care System.' *Canadian Journal of Public Health* 75 (January/February): 92–7

Pineault, Raynald, Andre-Pierre Contandriopoulos, and M.A. Fournier. 1985. 'Physician's Acceptance of an Alternative to Fee-for-Service Payment: A Possible Source of Change in Quebec Medicine.' *International Journal of Health Services* 15(3): 419–30

Pineault, Raynald, Andre-Pierre Contandriopoulos, and Richard Lessard. 1985. 'The Quebec Health System: Care Objectives or Health Objectives?' *Journal of Public Health Policy* 6(3): 394–409

Political Labor League. 1898. Fighting Platform, New South Wales

Polls, Vol. 1, no. 1, Spring 1965

Porter, John. 1965. *The Vertical Mosaic.* Toronto: University of Toronto Press

Porter, the Hon. J.R. 1985. Address to the State Conference, the Private Hospitals and Nursing Homes Association of Australia, Brisbane, 26 September

Preece, Rod. 1980. 'The Anglo-Saxon Conservative Tradition.' *Canadian Journal of Political Science* 13(1): 3–32

Pressman, Jeffrey L., and Aaron Wildavsky. 1973. *Implementation.* Berkeley: University of California Press

Progressive Conservative Party of Canada. n.d. *Campaign Handbook*

– n.d. 'A Brief History of the Progressive Conservative Party of Canada.' Typescript

Pross, Paul A., ed. 1975. *Pressure Group Behaviour in Canadian Politics.* Toronto: McGraw-Hill Ryerson

Pryor, Frederic L. 1968. *Public Expenditures in Communist and Capitalist Nations.*
London: George Allen and Unwin

Przeworski, A., and H. Teune. 1970. *The Logic of Comparative Social Enquiry.* New
York: Wiley Interscience

Queensland Labor Party. 1905. *Fighting Platform and General Programme,* May

Ray, John. 1975. 'Public Opinion Polls and Attitude Measurement.' *Current Affairs Bulletin* 52(2): 24–30

Reagan, M. 1972. *The New Federalism.* New York: Oxford University Press

Reeves, W.P. 1902. *State Experiments in Australia and New Zealand,* vol. 1. London:
Macmillan

*Report of the Commission of Enquiry into the Efficiency and Administration of Hospi-
tals.* 1981. (Jamison Enquiry), vols. 1 and 2. Canberra: AGPS

Report of the Commonwealth Committee of Enquiry. Health Insurance (Nimmo
Report). 1969. Canberra: Government Printer

Report of the Royal Commission on Health. 1926. Canberra: Government Printer
for the State of Victoria and the Government of the Commonwealth of Australia

'Report of the Social Security Medical Survey Committee,' Vol. 1, 1943. Canberra:
Typescript

Report on Health and Pensions Insurance (Kinnear Report). 1937. Canberra: Government Printer

Reports of the National Health and Medical Research Council, 11th Session July 1941,
12th Session November 1941, 14th Session November 1942, 16th Session December 1943, 17th Session May 1944, 18th Session November 1944

Richards, John, and Larry Pratt. 1979. *Prairie Capitalism.* Toronto: McClelland and
Stewart

Richter, Maxwell. 1986. 'A Doctor Looks at His Profession: What Went Wrong?'
CMA Journal 135 (1 September): 522–4

Riker, William H. 1969. 'Six Books in Search of a Subject or Does Federalism
Exist and Does It Matter?' *Comparative Politics* 2(1): 135–46

– 1970. 'The Triviality of Federalism.' *Politics* 5(2): 239–41

Roberts, David. 1969. *Victorian Origins of the Welfare State.* New Haven: Yale
University Press

Robin, R.D. 1966. 'The British Medical Association in Queensland.' BA thesis,
University of Queensland

Rodwin, Victor G. 1982. 'Management without Objectives: The French Health
Policy Gamble.' In Gordon McLachlan and Alan Maynard, eds., *The Public/Pri-
vate Mix for Health,* 289–325. London: Nuffield Provincial Hospitals Trust

– 1983. *The Health Planning Predicament: France, Quebec, England and the United
States.* Berkeley: University of California Press

Roe, Jill, ed. 1976. *Social Policy in Australia*. Stanmore: Cassell Australia

Roe, M. 1976. 'The Establishment of the Australian Department of Health: Its Background and Significance.' *Historical Studies* 17(67): 76–192

Romanow, Roy, John Whyte, and Howard Leeson. 1984. *Canada Notwithstanding*. Toronto: Carswell/Methuen

Russell, Peter H. 1985. 'The Supreme Court and Federal-Provincial Relations: The Political Use of Legal Resources.' *Canadian Public Policy* 11(2): 161–70

Sabetti, Fileppo, and Harold Waller. 1984. 'Introduction: Crisis and Continuity in Canadian Federalism.' *Publius* 14(1): 1–8

Sackville, Ronald. 1978. 'Social Welfare in Australia: The Constitutional Framework.' In Adam Graycar, ed., *Perspectives in Australian Social Policy*, 49–66. Melbourne: Macmillan

Saskatchewan Farmers Union. 1961. Presentation to the Advisory Planning Committee on Medical Care, January

Saskatchewan Federation of Labour. n.d. 'The First Fight for Medicare'

Saunders, Cheryl, and Kenneth Wiltshire. 1980. 'Fraser's New Federalism 1975–1980: An Evaluation.' *Australian Journal of Politics and History* 26(3): 355–71

Sawer, G. 1963. *Australian Federal Politics and Law 1929–1946*. London and New York: Cambridge University Press

– 1972. 'The Dynamics of Australian Federalism.' *Round Table* 62: 248, 441–50

– 1976. *Modern Federalism*. Carlton: Pitman Australia

– 1977a. *Australian Government Today*, 12th ed. Melbourne: Melbourne University Press

– 1977b. *Federation under Strain: Australia 1972–75*. Melbourne: Melbourne University Press

– 1977c. 'Seventy Five Years of Australian Federalism.' *Australian Journal of Public Administration* 36(1): 1–11

Sawer, Marian. 1981. 'Looking Backwards – The Liberal Party and Laissez-Faire Liberalism.' *Australian Quarterly* 53(3): 252–61

– ed. 1982. *Australia and the New Right*. Sydney: George Allen and Unwin

Sax, S. 1980. 'Community Health Developments in Australia.' *Public Health Reviews* 9(3–4): 269–99

– 1984. *A Strife of Interests*. Sydney: George Allen and Unwin

Schattschneider, E.E. 1952. 'Political Parties and the Public Interest.' *The Annals of the American Academy of Politics and Social Science* 280: 18–26

– 1957. 'Intensity, Visibility, Direction and Scope.' *American Political Science Review* 51(4): 933–42

Schultz, Richard, Orest Kruhlak, and John Terry, eds. 1979. *The Canadian Political Process*, 3rd ed. Toronto: Holt Rinehart and Winston

Scott, Frank R. 1977. *Essays on the Constitution*. Toronto: University of Toronto Press

Scott, Roger, ed. 1980. *Interest Groups and Public Policy*. Melbourne: Macmillan

Scott-Young, Margery. 1962. 'The Nationalisation of Medicine.' *MJA Supplement* 18 August: 21–8

Scotton, R.B. 1967. 'Voluntary Insurance and the Incidence of Hospital Costs.' *Australian Economic Papers* 6: 171–91

– 1968. 'Voluntary Health Insurance in Australia.' *Australian Economic Review* 2nd Quarter: 37–44

– 1977. 'Medibank 1976.' *Australian Economic Review* 1st Quarter: 23–35

– 1978. 'Health Services and the Public Sector.' In R.B. Scotton and Helen Ferber, eds., *Public Expenditures and Social Policy in Australia*, vol. 1, 1–37. Melbourne: Longman Cheshire

– 1980. 'Health Insurance: Medibank and After.' In R.B. Scotton and Helen Ferber, eds., *Public Expenditures and Social Policy in Australia*, vol. 2, 1–27. Melbourne: Longman Cheshire

Scotton, R.B., and J.S. Deeble. 1968. 'Compulsory Health Insurance for Australia.' *Australian Economic Review* 4th Quarter: 9–16

– 1969. 'The Nimmo Report.' *Economic Record* 45(11): 258–75

Scullin, the Hon. J.H. 1928. *Labor Policy for the Commonwealth*, 4 October, Richmond, Victoria

Shack, P. 1988. 'Medicare Update.' *Health Issues* 16 (December): 10

Shackleton, Doris. 1975. *Tommy Douglas*. Toronto: McClelland and Stewart

Sharman, G.C. 1975. 'Federalism and the Study of the Australian Political System.' *Australian Journal of Politics and History* 21(3): 11–24

Shea, Brian. 1970. 'The Organisation of Health and Medical Care Services in Australia – The State's Point of View.' In *The Delivery of Health Services in Australia*, 37–63. Chicago: American College of Hospital Administrators

Sheehan, Peter. 1980. *Crisis in Abundance*. Victoria: Penguin

Simeon, Richard. 1972. *Federal-Provincial Diplomacy*. Toronto: University of Toronto Press

– 1976a. 'Studying Public Policy.' *Canadian Journal of Political Science* 9(4): 548–80

– 1976b. 'The "Overload Thesis" and Canadian Government.' *Candian Public Policy* 11(4): 541–52

– 1977. 'Regionalism and Canadian Political Institutions.' In J. Peter Meekison, ed., *Canadian Federalism: Myth or Reality*, 292–303. Toronto: Methuen

Simerl, Loren M. 1982. 'Provincial Election Results.' In Paul W. Fox, ed., *Politics: Canada*, 5th ed., 655–93. Toronto: McGraw-Hill Ryerson

Smiley, D.V. 1963. *The Rowell-Sirois Report*, Book 1. Toronto: McClelland and Stewart

– 1965. 'The Two Themes of Canadian Federalism.' *Journal of Economics and Political Science* 31(1): 80–97

– 1980. *Canada in Question: Federalism in the 1980's*, 3rd ed. Toronto: McGraw-Hill Ryerson

– 1984. 'Public Sector Politics, Modernisation and Federalism: The Canadian and American Experiences.' *Publius* 14(1): 39–59

Smith, Jennifer. 1983. 'The Origins of Judicial Review in Canada.' *Canadian Journal of Political Science* 16(1): 115–133

Social Welfare Commission. 1975. *Annual Report*. Canberra: Federal Capital Press

Soderstrom, Lee. 1981. 'Extra-billing and Cost-sharing.' *Canadian Public Policy* 7(1): 103–18

Solomon, David. 1978. *Inside the Australian Parliament*. Sydney: George Allen and Unwin

– 1983. 'Constitution and Politics: Conflict Constrained.' In Jennifer Aldred and John Wilkes, eds., *A Fractured Federation? Australia in the 1980's*, 63–78. Sydney: George Allen and Unwin

Somers, Herman. 1975. 'Health and Public Policy.' *Inquiry* 12: 87–96

Sproule-Jones, M.H. 1975. *Public Choice and Federalism in Australia and Canada*, Research Monograph no. 11. Canberra: Centre for Research on Federal Financial Relations, Australian National University

– 1984. 'The Enduring Colony? Political Institutions and Political Science in Canada.' *Publius* 14(1): 93–108

Starr, Graeme. 1977. 'Federalism as a Political Issue: Australia's Two "New Federalisms."' *Publius* 7(1): 7–26

Starr, Paul. 1982. *The Social Transformation of American Medicine*. New York: Basic Books

Stein, Michael B. 1984. 'Canadian Constitutional Reform, 1927–1982: A Comparative Case Analysis over Time.' *Publius* 14(1): 121–39

Stevenson, Garth. 1979. *Unfulfilled Union*. Toronto: Gage

Stewart, Ian. 1980. 'Of Customs and Coalitions: The Formation of Canadian Federal Parliamentary Alliances.' *Canadian Journal of Political Science* 13(3): 451–79

Symons, T.H.B. 1982. 'Two Federations.' In R.L. Mathews, ed., *Public Policies in Two Federal Countries: Canada and Australia*, 10. Canberra: Centre for Research on Federal Financial Relations, Australian National University

Task Force on Coordinating Health Services in the Community. 1983. 'The Development of Community Based Services.' Government of New South Wales, Typescript held in the Department of Health Library, Canberra

Task Force on the Allocation of Health Care Resources. n.d. *Health: A Need for Redirection*. Report of a project funded by the Canadian Medical Association in 1983

Tatchell, Michael, ed. 1982. *Economics and Health: 1981*, Proceedings of the Third

Australian Conference of Health Economists, Health Research Paper, Technical Paper 6. Canberra: Australian National University

– ed. 1983. *Economics and Health: 1982*, Proceedings of the Fourth Australian Conference of Health Economists, Health Research Paper, Technical Paper 7. Canberra: Australian National University

– ed. 1984a. *Economics and Health: 1983*, Proceedings of the Fifth Australian Conference of Health Economists, Health Research Paper, Technical Paper 8. Canberra: Australian National University

– ed. 1984b. *Perspectives on Health Policy*, Proceedings of a Public Affairs Conference, Australian National University, 27–29 July 1982. Canberra: Health Economics Research Unit, Australian National University

Taylor, Charles. 1982. *Radical Tories*. Toronto: Anansi

Taylor, M.G. 1949. 'The Saskatchewan Hospital Services Plan,' University of California. Mimeographed for limited distribution by the Saskatchewan Health Services Planning Commission

– 1960. 'The Role of the Medical Profession in the Formulation and Execution of Public Policy.' *Canadian Journal of Economics and Political Science* 36(1): 108–27

– 1978. *Health Insurance and Canadian Public Policy*. Montreal and Kingston: McGill–Queen's University Press

– 1980. 'The Canadian Health Insurance Program.' In Carl A. Meilicke and Janet L. Storch, eds., *Perspectives on Canadian Health and Social Services Policy: History and Emerging Trends*, 183–97. Ann Arbor, MI: Health Administration Press

– 1989. 'The Canadian Health Care System 1974–1984.' In Robert G. Evans and Greg L. Stoddart, eds., *Medicare at Maturity*, 3–39. Calgary: University of Calgary Press

Teeple, Gary, ed. 1972. *Capitalism and the National Question in Canada*. Toronto: University of Toronto Press

Terris, Milton. 1978. 'The Three Worlds of Medical Care: Trends and Prospects.' *American Journal of Public Health* 68(11): 1125–31

Thame, C. 1974. 'Health and the State: The Development of Collective Responsibility for Health Care in the First Half of the Twentieth Century.' PhD thesis, Australian National University

Thorburn, Hugh, ed. 1967. *Party Politics in Canada*, 2nd ed. Scarborough: Prentice Hall

Tierney, Leonard. 1970. 'Social Policy.' In A.F. Davies and S. Encel, eds., *Australian Society*, 2nd ed. Melbourne: Cheshire

Tiver, P.G. 1978. *The Liberal Party*. Milton: Jacaranda Press

Townsend, P., and N. Davidson. 1982. *Inequalities in Health*. London: Penguin

Trent, Bill. 1984. 'Quebec's Struggle for Community-Based Medicine.' *CMA Journal* 130 (1 May): 1185–89

Trudeau, Pierre. 1968. 'The Practice and Theory of Federalism.' In Pierre Trudeau, *Federalism and the French Canadians*, 124–50. Toronto: Macmillan of Canada

Truman, Tom. 1968. 'A Scale for Measuring a Tory Streak in Canada and the United States.' *Canadian Journal of Political Science* 10(3): 597–612

Tucker, K.A., ed. 1977. *Economics of the Australian Service Sector*. London: Croom Helm

Tulloch, Patricia. 1978. 'Normative Theory and Social Policy.' *Australia and New Zealand Journal of Sociology* 14(1): 65–74

– 1979. *Poor Policies*. London: Croom Helm

Tuohy, Carolyn. 1988. 'Medicine and the State in Canada: The Extra-Billing Issue in Perspective.' *Canadian Journal of Political Science* 21(2): 267–96

– 1989a. 'Federalism and Canadian Health Policy.' In W. Chandler and C. Zollner, eds., *Challenges to Federalism in Canada and the Federal Republic of Germany*, 141–60. Kingston: Queen's University Institute of Intergovernmental Relations

– 1989b. 'Conflict and Accommodation in the Canadian Health Care System.' In Robert G. Evans and Greg L. Stoddart, eds., *Medicare at Maturity* , 393–434. Calgary: University of Calgary Press

Uldall, P. Robert. 1986. 'Bill 94 Threatens Quality of Ontario Medicine.' CMA *Journal* 134 (15 February): 396–9

Van Loon, R.J. 1979. 'Reforming Welfare in Canada.' *Public Policy* 27(4): 469–504

– 1980. 'From Shared Cost to Block Funding and Beyond.' In Carl A. Meilicke and Janet L. Storch, eds., *Perspectives on Canadian Health and Social Services Policy: History and Emerging Trends*, 342–66. Ann Arbor, MI: Health Administration Press

– 1989. 'Canadian Perspective: Learning from Our Experience.' In Robert G. Evans and Greg L. Stoddart, eds., *Medicare at Maturity*, 451–72. Calgary: University of Calgary Press

Van Loon, R.J., and Michael Whittington. 1981. *The Canadian Political System*, 3rd ed. Toronto: McGraw-Hill Ryerson

Vayda, Eugene, and Raisa Deber. 1984. 'The Canadian Health Care System: An Overview.' *Social Science and Medicine* 18(3): 191–7

Vladeck, Bruce. 1984. 'If the War of 1812 Had Come Out Differently, Would We Now have PPO's in Manitoba or Fights over Extra Billing in Mississippi?' In Robert G. Evans and Greg L. Stoddart, eds., *Medicare at Maturity*, 443–50. Calgary: University of Calgary Press

Walmsley, D.J. 1980. *Social Justice and Australian Federalism*. Armidale: University of New England

Warhurst, John. 1983. 'Canada's Intergovernmental Relations Specialists.' *Australian Journal of Public Administration* 42(4): 459–85

Watts, R. 1983. 'The Light on the Hill: The Origins of the Australian Welfare State 1935–45.' PhD thesis, University of Melbourne

Watts, R.L. 1982. 'The Historical Development of Canadian Federalism.' In R.L. Mathews, ed., *Public Policies in Two Federal Countries: Canada and Australia*, 13–26. Canberra: Centre for Research on Federal Financial Relations, Australian National University

Weller, G.R. 1974. 'Health Care and Medicare Policy in Ontario.' In G. Bruce Doern and V. Seymour Wilson, eds., *Issues in Canadian Public Policy*, 85–114. Toronto: Macmillan of Canada

– 1977. 'From "Pressure Group Politics" to the "Medical–Industrial Complex."' *Journal of Health Politics, Policy and Law* 1(4): 444–70

– 1980. 'The Determinants of Canadian Health Policy.' *Journal of Health Politics, Policy and Law* 5(3): 405–17

– 1981. 'The Delivery of Health Services in the Canadian North.' *Journal of Canadian Studies* 16(2): 69–79

Weller, Geoffrey R., and Pranal Manga. 1983. 'The Push for Reprivatization of Health Care Services in Canada, Britain and the United States.' *Journal of Health Politics, Policy and Law* 8(3): 495–517

Wettenhall, Roger. 1985. 'Lubricating a Federal System.' *Current Affairs Bulletin* 61(11): 28–35

Wheare, K.C. 1953. *Federal Government*, 3rd ed. London: Oxford University Press

White, W.L., R.H. Wagenbury, and R.C. Nelson. 1981. *Introduction to Canadian Politics and Government*, 3rd ed. Toronto: Holt Rinehart and Winston

Whitlam, the Hon. E.G. 1971. 'A New Federalism.' *Australian Quarterly* 43(3): 6–17

– 1972. Policy Statement. Canberra: Australian Labor Party

– 1974. Policy Speech, 24 April. Canberra: Australian Labor Party

– 1975a. *Campaign 1975: An Address to the Nation*, 24 November

– 1975b. 'People and Power – Community Participation in Federal Government.' *Australian Quarterly* 47(2): 36–43

– 1978. 'Reform During Recession: The Way Ahead.' T.J. Ryan Memorial Lecture, University of Queensland, 28 April

Whittington, Michael S., and Glen Williams, eds. 1981. *Canadian Politics in the 1980's*. Toronto: Methuen

Wier, Richard A. 1973. 'Federalism, Interest Groups and Parliamentary Government: The Canadian Medical Association.' *Journal of Commonwealth Political Studies* 11: 159–75

Wilber, Richard. 1969. *The Bennett Administration 1930–1935*. Canadian Historical Association Booklets. no. 24. Ottawa: Canadian Historical Association

Wildavsky, A. 1967. *American Federalism in Perspective*. Boston: Little, Brown

– 1974. *The Politics of the Budgetary Process,* 2nd ed. Boston: Little, Brown

Wilenski, Peter. 1983. 'Six States or Two Nations.' In Jennifer Aldred and John Wilkes, eds., *A Fractured Federation? Australia in the 1980's,* 79–102. Sydney: George Allen and Unwin

Wilensky, Harold L. 1965. *The Welfare State and Equality.* Berkeley: University of California Press

Willis, Evan. 1983. *Medical Dominance.* Sydney: George Allen and Unwin

Wiltshire, Kenneth. 1986. *Planning and Federalism.* St Lucia: University of Queensland Press

Woods, David. 1982. 'BCMA Calls for Crown Corporation to Run Hospitals.' *CMA Journal* 127 (15 July): 148–51

Woodsworth, David. 1980. 'A Response to Professor Finday's Paper.' *Canadian Journal of Social Work Education* 6(1): 148–51

Yelaja, Shankar A. 1978. *Canadian Social Policy.* Waterloo: Wilfred Laurier University Press

Young, R.A., Philippe Faucher, and Andre Blais. 1984. 'The Concept of Province-Building: A Critique.' *Canadian Journal of Political Science* 17(4): 783–818

Index